Valuing, Selling, and Closing the Medical Practice

Practice Success Series

Max Reiboldt, CPA

AMA
AMERICAN
MEDICAL
ASSOCIATION

Internet address: www.ama-assn.org

Additional copies of this book may be ordered by calling 800 621-8335 or from the secure AMA Web site at www.amabookstore.com. Refer to product number OP314611.

BQ13:11-P-098:10/11

Library of Congress Cataloging-in-Publication Data

Reiboldt, J. Max. Valuing, selling, and closing the medical practice / Max Reiboldt.

p. cm. -- (Practice success series)
Includes bibliographical references and index.
Summary: "This resourse provides in-depth information on the fundamentals of strategic practice management and future planning for the medical practice in the areas of selling, closing, and valuation"-- Provided by publisher.

ISBN 978-1-60359-607-7

1. Medicine--Practice--Valuation. 2. Medicine--Practice--Economic aspects. I. American Medical Association. II. Title.
R728.R4454 2012
610.68--dc23
2011036416

TABLE OF CONTENTS

PREFACE

With economic factors and federal legislation taking its toll on physicians and their desire to deliver health care, physicians are forced to make tough decisions unrelated to patient care. This book seeks to provide guidelines for those who are considering or have decided to sell or close their practice as it is now and making these choices informed decisions. This book is a comprehensive resource for physicians who seek to appraise the value of their practice and explore various dissolution considerations.

Whether contemplating a sell-out, a close-out, or assessing your market position, broadening your knowledge base of such options will better prepare you for appropriate career modifications. With the most current information in the medical practice marketplace, this book assists physicians in asking the appropriate questions and attaining answers to the vital areas of consideration for each aspect of the business side of practicing medicine.

This practical resource provides in-depth information on the fundamentals of strategic practice management and future planning for the medical practice in the areas of selling, closing, and valuation. Each area explores various phases and processes required in undertaking and finalizing each effort. Even medical students and physicians in residency programs will want to explore the content to grasp the scope of business aspects as they apply to the medical practice and the challenges for which they must prepare. The author and contributors, based on their many years of work with physicians and hospital networks, address the landscape of the current health care environment and project the prospective impact on medical practices, especially as physicians plan for the future and transition their practice into new business settings.

Applicable to any level of medical education or experience, this guide identifies and simplifies the physicians' options for making the best decisions available for their career as they head into this new world of health care.

ACKNOWLEDGMENTS

Books written by employees of the Coker Group are always touched by the many people both inside and outside of our organization. This work is no exception. First, we would like to give a special thanks to the contributions made by our fellow Coker family for their expertise on this project: Justin Chamblee, Cynthia Cox, Aimee Greeter, Deborah Hill, Craig Hunter, David Julian, Rick Langosch, Greg Mayfield, Greg Mertz, Will Melson, John Reiboldt, Mark Reiboldt, and Yong Zhang. In addition to our primary author, Max Reiboldt, we thank you for extending your knowledge from your many years of working with medical practices and physician networks.

Kay Stanley, who has contributed to Coker's 50-plus books since Coker's publishing initiative began in the early 1990s, has served as editor and project manager. Trish Hutcherson has served as project coordinator.

Last, we appreciate the confidence of Carol Brockman, American Medical Association continuity editor, in supporting this project and allowing us to expand the Practice Success Series.

ABOUT THE AUTHOR

Max Reiboldt, CPA, provides sound financial and strategic solutions to hospitals, medical practices, health systems, and other health care entities through keen analysis and problem solving. Working with organizations of all sizes, Reiboldt engages in consulting projects with organizations nationwide. His expertise encompasses employee and physician employment and compensation, physician/hospital affiliation initiatives, business and strategic planning, mergers and acquisitions, practice operational assessments, ancillary services development, physician hospital organization/ independent practice association/ management services organization development, practice appraisals, and negotiations for acquisitions and sales. He also performs financial analyses for health care entities as well as buy/sell agreements and planning arrangements for medical practices.

Max Reiboldt is president and chief executive officer of Coker Group and has led the firm's growth since the late 1990s to its position today as one of the leading health care consulting firms in the United States and abroad. He is a prolific author and accomplished public speaker on health care management topics.

Mr. Reiboldt has authored or contributed to many of Coker Group's 50-plus books. Recent titles include *Financial Management of the Veterinary Practice* (©2010, AAHA Press), *RVUs at Work: Relative Value Units in the Medical Practice* (©2010, Greenbranch Publishing), *Physician Entrepreneurs: Strength in Numbers-Consolidation and Collaboration Strategies to Grow Your Practice* (©2008, HealthLeaders Media), *Physician Entrepreneurs: Going Retail—Business Strategies to Grow Beyond Traditional Practice Models* (©2007, HealthLeaders Media), *Financial Management of the Medical Practice, Third Edition* (©2011, American Medical Association), and *Reimbursement Management: Improving the Success and Profitability of Your Practice* (©2011, American Medical Association).

A graduate of Harding University, Reiboldt is a licensed Certified Public Accountant in Georgia and Louisiana, and a member of the American Institute of Certified Public Accountants, Healthcare Financial Management Association, and American Society of Appraisers.

CONTRIBUTORS

Justin Chamblee, MAcc, CPA, is a senior manager at Coker Group. He works with clients in a variety of strategic and financial areas, mainly dealing with physician compensation and hospital-physician transactions. These include the development and redesign of physician compensation plans for private practices and hospital-employed settings, as well as providing guidance to hospitals, physicians, and legal counsel as to the appropriateness of transactions between a hospital and a physician.

Mr. Chamblee has been a major contributor to recent Coker publications, including *Financial Management of the Veterinary Practice* (©2010, AAHA Press), *RVUs at Work: Relative Value Units in the Medical Practice* (©2010, Greenbranch Publishing), *Physician Entrepreneurs: Strength in Numbers-Consolidation and Collaboration Strategies to Grow Your Practice* (©2008, HealthLeaders Media), *Physician Entrepreneurs: Going Retail—Business Strategies to Grow Beyond Traditional Practice Models* (©2007, HealthLeaders Media), *Financial Management of the Medical Practice, Third Edition,* (©2011, American Medical Association), and *Reimbursement Management: Improving the Success and Profitability of Your Practice* (©2011, American Medical Association). Mr. Chamblee holds a Bachelor of Business Administration in Accounting and a Master of Accounting from Abilene Christian University. He is a licensed Certified Public Accountant in Texas and is a member of the American Institute of Certified Public Accountants.

Cynthia Cox, MSM, CPC, a Senior Associate with Coker Group, has over 15 years of experience in health care and medical practice management, both in primary care and in multispecialty practices, gaining knowledge and experience in many areas of health care. Ms. Cox draws on her experience and skill in practice management to assist a diverse group of Coker's clients with myriad operational and financial issues, including operations, accounts receivables, revenue cycle analyses, merger assistance, physician education and training in coding compliance issues, coding analyses, medical chart audits, practice assessments, and interim management assignments. Previous positions on the payer side of insurance have given her priceless insight into collections and other insurance issues.

Ms. Cox graduated from Clayton College & State University, attaining a Bachelor of Science with a concentration in health care management. She went on to obtain a Master in Science Management with a concentration in health care management from Troy State University.

Ms. Cox is also a Certified Professional Coder and a Certified Patient Account Representative.

Aimee Greeter, MPH, is a manager in the financial services service line within Coker Group. She works on a variety of consulting projects, including financial consulting, hospital accounts, practice management initiatives, as well as research and writing for various client projects. In her most recent engagement, Ms. Greeter coordinated post-merger integration efforts for a faith-based hospital system, with a particular focus on human resources and supply chain management.

Ms. Greeter earned a Master of Public Health in Health Policy and Management from the Rollins School of Public Health at Emory University. Additionally, she was an honors graduate of Michigan State University, where she attained a Bachelor of Science in Human Biology.

Deborah B. Hill serves as a manager in the practice management area, responsible for managing the delivery of services to physicians, both through client hospitals and to individual practices. Her broad experience encompasses the following areas: billing management, network contract negotiations, referral resource network, coding and consulting services, coding compliance management, negotiation of vendor contracts, electronic medical record implementation, and provider enrollment and credentialing. Ms. Hill holds a Master of Business Administration in Health Care Administration and a Bachelor of Business Administration in Management. Additionally, she is a Certified Professional Coder by the American Academy of Professional Coders, and a Certified Medical Practice Executive by the American College of Medical Practice Executives.

Craig Hunter, senior vice president for Coker Group's business development, works with health systems, hospital-based networks, multi- and single-specialty groups, and independent practices, facilitating phases of integration and practice development, including mergers, strategic planning, management reviews, and negotiations. Mr. Hunter's focus encompasses network development, manpower plans, operational assessments, compensation plans, and medical staff surveys. Mr. Hunter provides integrated network services to hospitals and independent practices. He regularly conducts physician need and feasibility analyses for hospitals and private practices, involving staff planning and market analysis. Assignments entail physician contract preparation, analysis, and negotiations. Mr. Hunter also speaks frequently to health systems and physician executives, administrators, and other health care personnel, and is a published author on such practice management topics as compensation, integration, and physician recruitment and employment.

David Julian, CPA, is a manager with Coker Group and possesses over 20 years of experience in financial services. Mr. Julian has extensive experience in planning and implementing accounting policies and procedures. His robust background in accounting, financial analysis, and problem-solving gives him insight into the unique financial needs and goals of his clients. His myriad operational experiences provide leadership in the development and evaluation of short- and long-term strategic financial objectives. Mr. Julian has held a wide range of executive, financial, and operational responsibilities, including the development of annual budgets, cash flow projections, and developing, implementing, and maintaining job cost systems. Mr. Julian is a graduate of David Lipscomb University in Nashville, Tennessee, and a Certified Public Accountant in Georgia. He is a member of the American Institute of Certified Public Accountants and the Georgia Society of Certified Public Accountants.

Rick Langosch, a senior vice president, works with hospital clients to realize sustainable improvements at the organizational, departmental, and services level. Coker Group's Hospital Strategies consulting practice provides timely and responsive solutions to its hospital clients in service line analysis, staffing/productivity benchmarking and analysis, interim management, and recovery audit contractor readiness. A seasoned health care executive, with over 25 years of experience managing operations and finance in hospitals and physician practices, Mr. Langosch has held a wide range of financial, operational, and information technology responsibilities, including multi-hospital ownership and hospital senior management positions. He uses that experience to assist Coker clients in developing a specific implementation strategy that will produce improved performance and drive profitability for their organizations. Mr. Langosch is a graduate of Eastern Illinois University in Charleston, Illinois, and he is a Fellow with the Healthcare Financial Management Association. He is active with the Georgia Chapter of the Healthcare Financial Management Association.

Greg Mayfield, CPA, a manager in Coker's financial services service line, is an experienced leader, attorney, and business professional with excellent communication skills and a broad background in corporate law, financing transactions, real estate, banking, and regulatory matters. Some of the specific projects completed by Mr. Mayfield include fee fairness and subsidy opinions, valuations and appraisals, mergers and acquisitions, divestitures and carve outs, start-ups, turnaround assistance, and a variety of strategic planning initiatives. Mr. Mayfield holds a Bachelor of Science in Accounting from the University of Alabama, and is a graduate of George Washington University Law School in Washington, DC (Juris Doctor, with honors). He also completed the Executive Education Program on Corporate Governance, Leadership, and Change at Harvard Business School. Mr. Mayfield is a member of the State Bar of Georgia (1993) and of the American Health Lawyers Association, and is a Certified Public Accountant in Alabama.

Will Melson is a senior vice president with Coker Group, where his expertise encompasses operational improvement, change management, organizational design, cost containment, revenue enhancement, strategic planning, and informational technology planning for clients in all of the firm's core focus areas. Mr. Melson has more than 20 years of experience in corporate line management and management consulting. Mr. Melson's experience includes his role as principal at PricewaterhouseCoopers, where he executed numerous operations and integration engagements with Fortune 500 corporations. Mr. Melson started his private sector career at Procter & Gamble and was co-founding principal of the Broadwell Group, a boutique management advisory firm. During this time, he served as Chief Executive Officer of Lux Corp and was a trusted advisor to numerous senior executives at public and private companies. Mr. Melson holds a Bachelor of Arts in Electrical Engineering from Tennessee Technological University, as well as Master of Business Administration from the Fuqua School of Business at Duke University, graduating Summa Cum Laude and Fuqua Scholar.

John Reiboldt is a managing director with Coker Capital Advisors. Prior to co-founding Coker Capital Advisors, Mr. Reiboldt spent more than 10 years with Coker Group. During his tenure, Mr. Reiboldt founded the firm's financial services group, which provided mergers and acquisitions and strategic financial advisory services to the health care industry. While leading the financial services group, Mr. Reiboldt executed numerous transactions and advisory assignments across a wide variety of health care subsectors, both domestically and internationally. In addition to his role with Coker Capital Advisors, Mr. Reiboldt holds board seats and observation rights with several privately-held health care companies.

Mr. Reiboldt earned his Bachelor of Business Administration in Economics at the University of Mississippi and his Master of Business Administration with a concentration in Finance from The Robinson College of Business at Georgia State University. During his graduate and undergraduate studies, Mr. Reiboldt performed internships with Applied Financial Group, Inc, where he performed health care equity research; Nauset Biomedical Partners, LLC, a life sciences venture capital firm; and The Leadership Institute, a not-for-profit strategy group based in the greater Washington, DC, area.

Mark Reiboldt is a vice president at Coker Capital Advisors and Co-Leader of Coker Group's Financial Advisory Services group. Previously, Mr. Reiboldt was with Coker Group. During his tenure, Mr. Reiboldt executed numerous strategy, transaction, and strategic financial advisory assignments for the firm's clients. Prior to Coker Group, Mr. Reiboldt was with Trammell Crow Company, where he executed transactions for firms in the financial services and communications sectors. Previously, Mr. Reiboldt was a political advisor to numerous elected officials and candidates in Washington, DC, and throughout the United States. Mr. Reiboldt serves on the boards of numerous for-profit and not-for-profit organizations within health care and other sectors. He received a Bachelor of Arts in Political Science from Georgia State University and a Master of Science in Financial Economics from the University of London.

Yong Zhang, CPA, is a manager with Coker Capital Advisors. Prior to joining Coker Capital Advisors, Ms. Zhang spent four years with Coker Group. During her tenure with Coker Group, Ms. Zhang worked for the firm's financial services group, where she assisted in mergers and acquisitions, valuations and fairness opinions, and numerous advisory assignments across a wide spectrum of health care subsectors. Ms. Zhang earned her Bachelor of Accounting at Fudan University in Shanghai, China, and her Master of Accountancy from the University of Georgia. Prior to her position at Coker Group, Ms. Zhang was an accountant at General Motors of China. Ms. Zhang is a Certified Public Accountant in Georgia and is in the process of completing her Accredited Senior Appraiser designation. Ms. Zhang is fluent in Chinese.

ABOUT COKER GROUP

Coker Group, a leader in health care consulting, helps providers achieve improved financial and operational results through sound business principles. The consulting team members are proficient, trustworthy professionals with expertise and strengths in various areas. Coker Group represents four service lines: Coker Consulting, Coker Capital Advisors, Coker Technology, and Executive Search. Through these service areas, Coker consultants enable providers to concentrate on patient care.

Coker Group's nationwide client base includes major health systems, hospitals, physician and specialty groups, and solo practitioners in a full spectrum of engagements. Since 1987, Coker Group has gained a reputation for thorough, efficient, and cost-conscious work to benefit its clients financially and operationally. The firm prides itself on its client profile of recognized and respected health care professionals through the industry. The firm's exceptional consulting team has health care, technical, financial, and business knowledge and offers comprehensive programs, services, and training to yield long-term solutions and turnarounds. Coker staff members are devoted to helping health care providers face today's challenges for tomorrow's successes.

Service areas include:

- Capital advisory and strategic financial advisory and analysis
- Strategic planning/business planning
- Accountable care organization readiness
- Practice operational assessments
- Physician network development
- Disengagements of practices and network unwinds
- Hospital-physician alignment
- Practice management, billing and collections reviews, chart audits
- Compensation
- Post-merger integration implementation
- Hospital services, medical staff development
- Executive search
- Interim and long-term network management

- Practice appraisals
- Practice start-ups
- Buy/sell and equity analysis
- Group formation and dissolution
- Practice acquisition, mergers, and due diligence
- Compensation reviews, fair market value opinion services, and call coverage compensation
- *Health Insurance Portability and Accountability Act* assessments and compliance
- Market service agreement development
- Revenue cycle management and procedural coding analysis
- Compliance plans
- Policy and procedure manuals
- Mediation and expert witnessing
- Strategic information technology planning and review, including electronic health records
- HIT software/hardware vendor vetting and procurement
- Contract negotiations
- Project management
- Managed information technology services
- Educational programs, workshops, and training

For more information, please contact:

Coker Group
1000 Mansell Exchange West
Suite 310
Alpharetta, GA 30022
800-345-5829
www.cokergroup.com

PART ONE

Selling the Medical Practice

Valuing, Selling, and Closing the Medical Practice begins with preparing to sell, explores initiatives for enhancing the value of the practice, and addresses the processes and phases of disengagement. Chapters 1 through 4 cover marketing strategies for selling, seeking professional assistance, physician diversification, and practice buy-in/buyout.

CHAPTER 1
Practice Sale

OUTLINE

I. Introduction
II. Preparing for Selling
   A. Assessing Market Position
      1. Competition
      2. Payer Mix Variation
      3. General Economic Conditions
      4. Supply and Demand
      5. Substitution
      6. The Human Element
      7. Other Forces
   B. Value Enhancement Initiatives
   C. Maximizing Revenue
      1. Payment Strategies
      2. Medicare Payment Strategies
      3. Relative Value Units
      4. Accountable Care Organizations (ACO) and Patient-Centered Medical Homes
      5. Managed Care Implications
      6. Managing the Revenue Cycle
   D. Expense Control
      1. Internal Controls
         a. Safeguarding Cash
         b. Safeguarding Various Assets
         c. Personnel Policies and Procedures
      2. Expenditure Controls
         a. Practice Operating Overhead
         b. Fixed vs Variable Expenses
         c. Physician Compensation and Benefits

        d. Enhanced Quality
        e. ACO Development
- III. Marketing Strategies for Selling
    - A. Identifying Prospective Purchasers
        1. Outside Investors, Insurance Companies, and Health Maintenance Organizations
        2. Private Practicing Physicians
    - B. Consultants/Attorneys
    - C. Other Ways to Purchase or Sell a Practice
        1. Networking
        2. Advertising
- IV. Professional Assistance
    - A. The Attorney
    - B. The Accountant
    - C. The Broker
    - D. The Consultant
- V. Governance
- VI. Unwind Provisions
- VII. Dissolution
    - A. Cash, Equivalents, and Other Assets
    - B. Accounts Receivable
    - C. Accounts Payable
    - D. Tax Considerations
        1. Property Taxes
        2. Payroll Taxes
        3. Sales Taxes/Local Taxes
        4. Income/Franchise Taxes
    - E. Legal Entity Termination
- VIII. Transitioning to the New Owner
    - A. Patients
    - B. Managed Care Organizations
    - C. Personnel
        1. Employee Hiring and Firing
        2. Record Keeping
        3. Health Insurance Benefits
        4. Other Benefits
        5. Medical Records
    - D. The Phase-Out Agreement
- IX. Conclusion

The sale of a medical practice demands serious contemplation over an extended period. Ample time is needed to address all the considerations and complete the entire continuum of work. This continuum includes due diligence, valuation, marketing, actual identification of a potential buyer through the agreement process, and, ultimately, the dissolution and transitioning processes. Figure 1-1 illustrates the continuum of work that is required from the beginning to the end of this process.

During the late 1990s and the early 2000s, the number of physicians selling practices decreased, primarily because the market for buying practices became smaller. Now, within the industry, the pace of sales has picked up considerably for both primary care and specialty practices. Specialties that previously would not have considered selling and becoming employees or partners of a larger group or health system or hospital are now in the market. Clearly, the market has changed relative to the value of practices, in that little or no goodwill or intangible asset value is being paid, especially if it is to another group through a type of merger or to a health system. Most acquirers, especially hospitals, are only paying for the tangible asset value of the practice; any potential intangible value that otherwise would have been considered is attributable to the compensation structure over the subsequent period of employment. Although this chapter does not focus on the dynamics relative to the marketplace or on valuation methodologies, it does consider appropriate scenarios for selling practices and strategies for completing this important process.

Physicians deserve to receive fair market value for what they have created through diligence and dedication in building a stable base of revenue and management infrastructure. However, fair market value in the truest sense is also changing, consistent with the types of transactions, as discussed. To attain fair value for a practice, whether that value payment is evident in the tangible assets, in the unlikely occurrence of some intangible asset value, or via a fair market value or commercially reasonable compensation structure going forward, the practice must be open to review, due diligence, and scrutiny by the prospective purchaser.

It is important for the selling physicians to obtain competent professional assistance from both outside consultants and legal counsel. These individuals should understand both the valuation and sales process. Moreover, they should be savvy as to the types of transactions that are occurring in the industry and the methodologies of structure surrounding the sales. (For example, they should know that now, most of the "value" is tied to the compensation of the physicians going forward.)

Sellers who seek to retire also must understand the current market trends and adjust accordingly; likewise, not looking for significant intangible value. However, if they do not plan to be employed, some possibilities of additional value may be tied to intangible assets within that practice sale.

Sellers of practices should understand and identify the reasons for selling. Moreover, they must prepare the practice for sale and develop

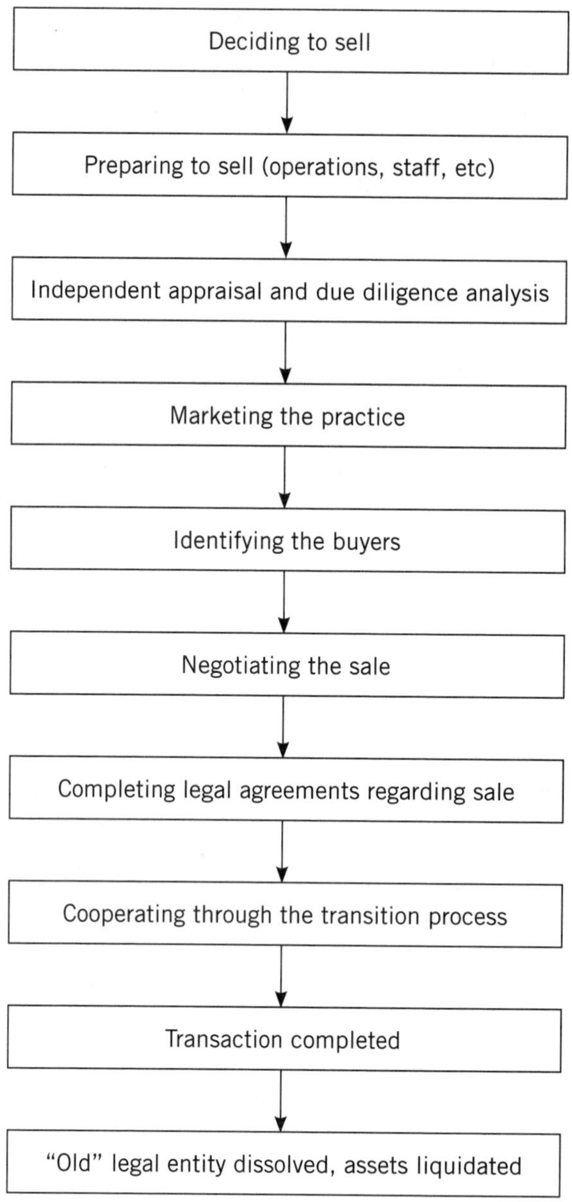

FIGURE 1-1 Continuum of Work

market strategies to receive optimal value, within legal and regulatory parameters. Proper planning will result in substantiated legal documentation and, after the sale, a plan of transition and/or dissolution of the practice, as applicable, should be in place. Considerations for selling a practice are discussed in Chapter 5; dissolution matters are discussed in Chapter 6.

Preparing for Selling

Although the market has changed, the sale of the practice requires adequate preparation. The primary goal of any sale is to attain maximum value, regardless of the purpose of the sale, even if the sellers continue as employees or partners after the sale or totally sell and leave the market to retire or for other pursuits. The initial basis for negotiating the sales price is indeed the valuation. However, before the appraiser performs the valuation (or perhaps during its completion), much can be done to enhance the value of a practice.

Assessing Market Position

The first step is to analyze the practice's market position by examining the practice's relationship to national, regional, and local economies. Also, its position is reviewed within the specific profession. Sources of information include the following:

- Market analysis
- Feasibility study
- Study of principles that influence values (eg, supply and demand, competition, changing conditions)
- Research of industry trends

An understanding of the local marketplace is important to prospective sellers. Important components must be considered, and a discussion of each follows.

Competition

The professional medical practice is a business with competitors nearby. It is conceivable (and likely) that the practice being sold is similar to other practices in a local area. This varies, however, with population centers. For example, in rural areas where medical practices are scarce, competition is minimal. Demand increases value in areas where limited or no competition exists.

Payer Mix Variation

Payer mix significantly influences the assessment of market conditions of the practice. If the patient population is covered by Medicare and Medicaid, significant discounting of fees can be expected (but may be offset by a higher volume of patients). In an environment in which managed care is prevalent, fees are either discounted or capitated. In a more traditional, fee-for-service patient population, the fee structure will yield a more lucrative practice and result in a higher value and sales price. The practice sale also must be considered in the context of payment systems such as accountable care organizations (ACO), as ACOs become a part of the payment landscape.

General Economic Conditions

Economic conditions, including general health care supply and demand, affect practice values and ultimately the sales price. Trends in population, employment, and income are continually changing and influencing economic stability. Economic conditions also affect a practice's ability to expand; likewise, they affect the sellers' ability to obtain an acceptable sales price. Conditions such as these have largely caused the emphasis away from significant upfront value tied to intangible assets. Current trends can be researched by asking the following questions: Is the practice in a growing community? Are people leaving the area? What is the local industry and is it growing? What are the ages of the residents? What is the unemployment rate? (It can be very significant if a manufacturing plant closes and the unemployed workers have no health care coverage.) How many new jobs were created in the last year? These indicators influence general economic conditions and, ultimately, the sale of the practice.

Supply and Demand

A basic economic principle that applies to all industries, including health care, is supply and demand. The value of a practice is influenced by the number of buyers available compared with the number of practices for sale. To evaluate this, first determine whether it is a buyer's or a seller's market. If many similar practices are on the market or if the demand for them is declining, it is a buyer's market and the sales price of a practice will be reduced. Conversely, if demand for a certain type of specialty practice increases and supply remains constant (ie, no new practices of this type are opening), the price for that specialty practice should increase.

In general, the demand for established practices in most areas of the country has grown rapidly as health care continues to transition. Due to increased costs, the number of group practices is on the rise, and solo practices are diminishing in quantity. Physicians entering private practice are either purchasing existing businesses from their retiring colleagues, moving, or shifting to employed (salaried) positions. In addition, practices are operated as competitive businesses. Once again, demand has increased as hospitals have started buying and owning medical practices. However, because the industry trend in response to a changing payment paradigm is to form integrated delivery systems, this demand has not translated into significant upfront value. Most selling physicians must accept that the economics have changed even though demand is considerably increased.

Substitution

The economic principle of substitution assumes that buyers will not pay the asking price of a particular practice when another equally desirable available practice is producing similar returns with comparable risk. When making an offer on an existing practice, prospective purchasers should base the offer on recent selling prices of comparable practices and on the expected return on investment. From the sellers' view, acceptance of an offer depends on two items: (1) the minimum amount that buyers could purchase an equally desirable practice and (2) the least amount sellers are willing to accept for that practice. This second point is influenced by the acceptable options available if sellers refuse to sell. Again, with hospitals returning to purchasing practices and employing physicians, there is a pent-up demand; however, this time the structures of the acquisitions rarely result in a significant windfall purchase price.

The Human Element

Emotion comes into play in the sale of a medical practice (perhaps more than in any other type of buying and selling transaction). Practicing medicine entails more than holding a job. Medicine is a way of life, driven by a desire to improve the quality of life and to help the ill become well. Most physicians are profoundly dedicated to their profession. As a seller, physicians often view the practice as the outcome of years of hard work and dedication. Deciding to sell is a traumatic event, and transitioning to another form of ownership or employment produces conflicting emotions. Although emotion does not alter the objective value of the practice, it does affect the owner's perception of value. Emotion can play an even greater role when physicians do not intend to continue in the practice and want to impart the new owner with the same care and concern for the patients in that practice. Finally, the emotion of selling to a health system or hospital carries the desire for a continued role in governance and operations. The new employer-owner may allow this participation, depending on the individual situation and the policy of the health system or hospital.

Other Forces

Social, political, legal, and governmental factors influence practice value. State and federal statutes along with professional ethical standards regulate the organization of a medical practice and restrict the private practice ownership to specified licensed practitioners (if it is to continue as a "professional" designated entity and/or if the state disallows the corporate practice of medicine). These elements significantly limit the marketplace, although generally the issues inhibiting such ownership can be mitigated relatively easily.

Value Enhancement Initiatives

For an owner, achieving optimum value is both legal and proper. The owner has the right to do whatever is legally justifiable to maximize the selling price of the practice, providing no financial manipulations occur. (Note: Today, maximizing "value" may well be accomplished through a better [ie, larger] compensation package post-transaction, assuming the owner physician will continue with the practice as an employee.) Likewise, the prudent buyer will perform all the necessary analyses and due diligence before making an acquisition.

By applying sound business practices, the owner will produce better operating results and will yield a higher sales price for the practice, making it more attractive to a prospective buyer. Although the following steps are a part of everyday operations, they are especially important in preparing a practice to sell. Key steps to take include:

- Maximizing revenue
  - Payer mix
  - Payment strategies
  - Managed care implications
  - Increasing productivity (both in collections and work-only relative value units [wRVU])
- Developing sound internal controls
  - Safeguarding cash
  - Safeguarding miscellaneous assets
  - Implementing fair personnel policies and procedures
- Controlling expenses
  - Practice operational overhead
  - Physician compensation and benefits
- Enhanced quality
  - Physicians quality reporting system
  - Pay-for-performance and other quality-related programs sponsored by private payers
  - Accountable care development
    - Accountable care organization (ACO) participation

- Patient-centered medical home involvement
- National Committee for Quality Assurance (NCQA) and similar accreditation and credentialing programs

Maximizing Revenue

Managing the medical practice to a point that revenue is maximized is a tremendous challenge in today's environment. This management process should be broken down into the revenue cycle. The cycle is a continuous process that must be efficiently completed. If it is not completed, a reduction in revenue is likely to occur. There are both internal and external factors that influence the revenue cycle; several of these will be described.

The payer mix, which is vital to maximizing revenue in preparation to sell a practice, identifies the makeup of payers in the practice, eg, patient self-pay, traditional or indemnity insurance, managed care (capitated and fee-for-service), Medicare, and Medicaid. Depending on the type of practice, the payer mix can cause operating results to vary significantly. For example, a practice based heavily on Medicare patients will receive payments for professional fees that are substantially discounted from the normal fee schedule. In most locations, this practice will have lower profit margins than a practice with a more varied payer mix and fewer contractual discounts (ie, a practice that is more traditional fee-for-service). However, Medicare patients are usually sicker and need more services and tests, which can increase the revenue per patient visit.

A practice containing many Medicaid patients is even more detrimental to profit margins. Also, payment through health savings accounts and other high-deductible plans can result in higher levels of uncollectible accounts. The strategy should be to avoid unacceptable payer mixes. Evaluate the following elements when determining payer mix:

- Age of the physicians and their practice
- Age of the physicians' patients
- Strategic alliances as a source for patient referrals
- Marketing strategies for the practice
- Managed care involvement
- Geographic setting (urban versus rural)
- Average collectible billing per patient visit

Begin to monitor these trends long before deciding to sell, and undertake initiatives for change. Of course, this is easier said than done and is even more difficult for some specialties. For example, an internist will find it difficult to avoid seeing Medicare patients, so non-Medicare patients must be added to change the mix. Developing a balanced payer mix enhances practice value and increases the sales price.

Payment Strategies

Obtaining maximum payment from payers is fundamental to securing the long-term economic viability of the practice. It is critical to set professional fees that will ultimately result in actual collections. The goal of every medical practice is to set reasonable and fair fees for all services that exceed what third-party payers reimburse. If the fee schedule can be legitimately set to obtain maximum payment, collections will be enhanced, earnings will be increased, and the practice will yield higher proceeds when sold (perhaps in the compensation package going forward, if not in an upfront payout).

In preparation for selling the practice (and for maximizing payment), regularly analyze fees. This analysis can be done by your practice administrator or a consultant. Sophisticated methods are used to review fee schedules and compare them with allowable payments for all types of payers. Payers include government and private payers such as insurance or managed care companies. A good starting place is to review insurance explanation of benefits (EOB) statements; retrieving an actual EOB and reviewing its reimbursement in relation to the practice's fee schedule is an easy, yet beneficial exercise.

The EOB shows how much the physician has billed and how much the insurance company has approved for payment. The copayments and deductible owed by the patient should be considered here as well. To assess the viability of professional fees relating to commercial insurance companies, review each Current Procedural Terminology (CPT®) code. If an insurer is paying 100% of current fees (less deductible amounts), an opportunity likely exists for additional payment and increased collections.

Medicare Payment Strategies

In 1992, the federal agency that controls Medicare payment levels developed a new prospective payment system for Medicare Part B. This system was adopted by the Centers for Medicare and Medicaid Services (CMS), formerly the Health Care Financing Administration (HCFA). At that time, managed care was in an earlier stage of implementation (even though managed care technically began in the 1970s), and the Medicare program was not under the current cost control measures. Little information regarding reimbursement rates was available from third-party payers. As a result, CMS concluded that third-party carriers operated under what was known as a "nondisclosed" maximum allowable policy.

Although a predetermined maximum amount allocated to each CPT code had been set, insurers did not provide that information to physicians. Providers did not know the amounts of maximum allowable payment that were determined to be reasonable and customary in their geographic areas for third-party carriers. As a result, a new approach to fee scheduling and revenue optimization for payers of Medicare payment was developed. Today, physicians should compare individual Medicare CPT code payment with their own private fee schedule to measure the impact of Medicare on the practice's revenue. This exercise is especially important, because most managed care organizations now reimburse on the basis of a Medicare multiple.

Relative Value Units

A readily accepted methodology for measuring physician productivity is the relative value unit (RVU), specifically the work-only RVU (wRVU). Under the fee schedule payment system, payment rates are based on relative weights. These account for the relative costliness of the inputs used to provide physician services: physician work, practice expenses, and professional liability insurance (PLI) expenses. The RVUs for physicians' work reflect the relative levels of time, effort, skill, and stress associated with providing each service. At least every five years, the fee schedule's relative weights are updated; Healthcare Common Procedure Coding System (HCPCS) codes and the conversion factor are updated annually. The update of relative weights includes a review of changes in medical practice, coding changes, new data, and the addition of new services. In completing its review, CMS receives advice from a group of physicians and other professionals sponsored by the American Medical Association and physician specialty societies.[1]

The RVU has become a primary way of evaluating physician productivity because they are "payer blind." As such, the productivity metric is not dependent on the actual dollars charged or ultimately collected. This system creates a standardization of productivity and a way to measure that productivity in the context of physician specialties. Moreover, RVUs (and especially wRVUs) are benchmarks; they become a major source of determining practice performance and physician productivity.

In the context of a practice sale, RVUs are a major way of evaluating performance, in particular, physician productivity. Hospitals will often use RVUs as a methodology for physician compensation. This use means that after the sale of the practice and subsequent employment of the physician by the health system or hospital, RVUs become the basic measure of productivity, with compensation derived from a conversion factor (sometimes called a multiplier). The conversion factor is multiplied by the total number of wRVUs to derive compensation. (Although an oversimplification of the compensation structure, this explanation illustrates the point within the context of this discussion.)

Thus, RVUs become a significant part of the overall due diligence and measurement of performance in the context of the practice sale.

Accountable Care Organizations and Patient-Centered Medical Homes

In addition to the other basic areas of consideration relative to revenue and payment, a new dynamic is occurring. Accountable care organizations (ACO) and patient-centered medical homes (PCMH) are becoming a part of the payment paradigm. An ACO is an organization of health care providers that agrees to be accountable for the quality, cost, and overall care of Medicare beneficiaries who are enrolled in the traditional fee-for-service program and who are assigned to that ACO.[2] The PCMH "is an approach to providing comprehensive primary care for children, youth, and adults in a health care setting that facilitates partnerships between individual patients, their personal clinicians, and, when appropriate, the patient's family."[3]

Medicare is introducing many changes in the payment paradigm, such as the Medicare Shared Savings Program: Accountable Care Organizations. Although the need for widespread participation seemed likely when first announced by CMS, the push toward this payment methodology has mellowed somewhat with the recent release of Proposed Rules. After a comment period that ended June 6, 2011, more direction will likely emerge regarding the impact of ACOs.

Commercial payers customarily follow the steps taken by Medicare. Although not moving totally away from fee-for-service payment, the emphasis is increasingly on quality and cost containment. In January 2012, Medicare expects to start sharing savings (and, in some cases, losses) based on these measurements of performance as opposed to direct productivity. Again, private insurers are already initiating such programs, with more expected. The physician whose practice is preparing for sale, therefore, must have a plan and be able to demonstrate that the practice performs at high levels of quality outcomes and has the ability to control costs. Moreover, this entire situation is driving consolidation.

The concept of bundled payments is being considered by payers and likely will become a part of the payment structure for Medicare. Private payers are expected to follow. This concept simply means that the payer will issue one payment for the continuum of care, and all providers, including hospitals and physicians (and perhaps others such as diagnostic, rehabilitation, and ancillary service providers) must decide how that bundled payment will be distributed to their individual entities. If these provider entities are consolidated into one organization, it will be easier to determine the allocation from the bundled payment.

For more information concerning ACOs and PCMHs, readers should consult recently published proposed regulations and other resources. ACOs are still very new; CMS has not fully documented its requirements, and regulations that provide guidance have just been issued. Regardless, for physicians preparing to sell a practice, it will be essential to consider quality, cost containment, and the new payment paradigms that will result. In fact, in many instances, these are the primary drivers why physicians are selling their practices and becoming employed by health systems or hospitals.

Managed Care Implications

Managed care is described as a system of health care services provided and financed to a specific group of recipients. Managed care plans involve alliances or contractual relationships of health care providers intended to produce the following results:

- Reduce health care costs
- Encourage preventive health care
- Effectively utilize health care resources

The best-known managed care products are preferred provider organizations (PPO) and health maintenance organizations (HMO), although there are numerous variations. Also, health savings accounts, health retirement accounts, and high-deductible plans have become far more prevalent in the last decade. However, the landscape is changing, as the concepts of accountable care are tied more to quality payments and shared cost savings.

Most health care providers agree that the shift within the industry toward managed care has caused providers to:

- Have an advantage participating in larger practice-contracting structures
- Be forced to participate in integrated delivery systems
- In a few locations, become employees for HMOs

Now, as the industry, led by CMS and several prominent insurance companies, shifts from managed care to accountable care, the emphasis on payment is not limited to a fee-for-service or a capitated payment structure.

This shift in managed care has created great apprehension among physicians and has influenced the numbers and prices of practices sold. This trend is especially true as hospitals and physicians are aligning in unprecedented numbers as a result of the Patient Protection and Affordable Care Act (PPACA) of 2010. When preparing to sell the practice, the physician should consider the impact of managed and accountable care not only for today but also for the future. By positioning the practice for the increased involvement of managed and accountable care in the future, sellers will enhance the attractiveness of the practice to prospective buyers.

Managing the Revenue Cycle

Proper management and supervision of the revenue cycle includes the internal revenue cycle as well as the external revenue cycle. Figure 1-2 illustrates the key components of both of these revenue cycles.

Physicians who have an understanding of each of these areas of operation, all of which contribute to an effective and efficient payment strategy, will be better prepared not only to sell the practice but also to enhance its value.

Influences on the external revenue cycle must also be considered, including the implications of managed care as well as governmental regulations. The requirement to be in compliance is seemingly of greater

General Revenue Cycle

- Most important source for improving financial performance
- External
  - Managed care
  - Federal regulation
- Internal
  - Controlled by practice
  - Typically may result in 5% to 15% increase in net collections

External Revenue Cycle

Payer Trends

- Converting to payment-based fixed-fee schedule
- Reducing fee schedules; no annual increases
- Denial and/or bundling of claims to reduce payments
- Slowing the payment cycle

Federal Legislation

- Compliance related to fraud and abuse requirements
- Legislation creating administrative "savings" through standardization
- Health Insurance Portability and Accountability Act legislation requiring patient confidentiality

Controllable Components of Internal Revenue Cycle

- Patient scheduling/registration
- Eligibility verification/care authorization
- Financial counseling
- Charge capture
- Pricing and managed care fees
- Coding
- Utilization review
- Medical records
- Claims submission
- Third-party follow-up and collection
- Private pay and balance after insurance follow-up and collection
- Rejection processing
- Payment posting and verification
- Credit balance adjudication
- Appeals
- Managed care strategy and administration

FIGURE 1-2 Internal and External Revenue Cycles

significance than ever. New laws are being implemented that require the practice to have defined policies and procedures, including a written compliance plan, to ensure this compliance. With regulations from the 1996 Health Insurance Portability and Accountability Act (HIPAA) in effect and ACO requirements about to be implemented, compliance with federal and state regulations is even more important to assure a sound and effective practice operation.

Expense Control

Expense control can be separated into two categories: (1) internal controls that safeguard the handling of cash and (2) controls that guard the way funds are expended. With accountable care being a major new factor of the payment paradigm, expense savings across the entire health care delivery system will become an even greater area of importance relative to the marketability and value of a practice for sale. Following are overviews of ways of handling each category of controls.

Internal Controls

Practices should have internal controls in place to prevent or minimize the risk of embezzlement or other office thievery or misuse. These processes, when implemented, enhance the stability and value of the entity. Although basic to any business, the ability to demonstrate such controls through policies, procedures, and processes, plus adequate numbers of qualified staff, enhances the practice's potential in a sale.

Safeguarding Cash. Instituting sound internal controls begins with the safeguarding of cash, which is fundamental to obtaining a maximum sales price. Although most medical practices handle very little cash, opportunities still arise for staff members to misappropriate monies and engage in unauthorized activity. Internal controls, when initiated, will reduce the likelihood for illicit activities to occur. Because most medical practices use a cash-based accounting method, ie, they recognize revenue when money is collected and expenses when payment is made, it is essential to ensure that the fees billed, after discounts and contractual allowances are applied, are collected. Fees become revenue when monies are deposited into the practice's bank account; billing is only an estimate of revenue. When accounts receivable are included in the sales price, they too can be protected. Value increases if refunds are done properly and without illicit activity. Value also increases when accounts are tracked regularly to maximize collection.

Safeguarding Various Assets. Other tangible assets can be safeguarded by protecting and extending their life and usefulness, and thus protecting their value. Maintaining equipment in good condition is less expensive than losing revenue because a piece of equipment is not working. Finally, controlling the payment for purchases of all types by implementing a sound approval process for accounts payable is fundamental to safeguarding the practice's assets.

Personnel Policies and Procedures. Value is enhanced when good personnel policies and procedures and effective internal controls are in place. Every practice should have a manual of personnel policies and procedures that documents personnel policies, benefits, and employee protocols. (Additional resources concerning the development of personnel policies and procedures can be found in Appendix A.)

Expenditure Controls

In conjunction with maximizing revenue, a medical practice's value is enhanced through the implementation of sound and functional cost controls. Some areas of expenses are more easily contained than others. The distinction between the types of expenses is explained in the following sections.

Practice Operating Overhead. In conjunction with maximizing revenue, a medical practice's value is enhanced through sound and functional cost controls. Both clinical and administrative functions generate practice overhead. For this reason, all functions should be monitored using a systematic review and approval of expenditures. Historical data of expenses can be captured using a basic medical practice statistical report.

Use summary information to analyze the practice's clinical activities, production, collections, contractual adjustments, and accounts receivable. Prepare and review these data monthly, and use the report for making management decisions and adjustments. These reports become even more vital when the practice is being prepared for sale. Following is a list of expenses to control:

- Adequate number of personnel
- Appropriate compensation levels for personnel
- Health insurance and other benefits (direct cost)
    - Overtime and retirement plan benefits (indirect cost)
    - Sick leave policy
    - Bereavement pay
    - Vacation
- Cost of medical supplies
- Cost of office supplies
- Lease and real estate arrangements
- Refunds to patients
- Advertising expense

- Professional fees, including billing and collection services
- Utilities
- Postage and other shipping charges
- Telephone expenses
- Smaller overhead items (eg, bank service charges, break room supplies)

Examine each expense to see if it is necessary for the efficient operation of the practice or simply for the owner's convenience. Eliminate convenience items to obtain a more accurate picture of how the practice is doing economically.

Memberships in professional medical practice management associations, such as the Medical Group Management Association (MGMA) and the American Medical Group Association (AMGA), and in state medical management associations can be helpful for learning what other practices are doing regarding costs control and revenue enhancement.

Fixed vs Variable Expenses. It is important to distinguish between fixed and variable expenses. In the most simplistic terms, fixed expenses are those that do not change with volume or revenue changes. Variable expenses are those that do change. Typically in the medical practice, the most common fixed expense is salaries (this could be semi-fixed or semi-variable for obvious reasons). Variable expenses would include such items as medical and office supplies, which change with fluctuations in revenue.

An extensive review of expenses is not provided here. However, it is important to note that most expenses in the medical practice are fixed or semi fixed. This feature actually has both a positive and a negative quality. The fact that most expenses are fixed makes them easier to control. However, the fact that most expenses are fixed also means that the total is going to be somewhat "fixed," making it difficult to reduce expenses. To solve this problem, you can increase revenue and maximize margins incrementally. As the margins increase with each additional dollar of revenue, those fixed or mostly fixed expenses will be covered. This relationship is illustrated in Figure 1-3.

The figure shows that with each additional dollar of revenue gained, profits are incrementally increased because most expenses are unchanged, albeit fixed. This process applies to both the general operations of the practice as well as the preparations to sell the practice. If prospective buyers of the practice can visualize opportunities to increase revenue while controlling expenses (again mostly fixed), the profits can be marginally improved.

Physician Compensation and Benefits. Physician compensation and benefits make up the other major portion of practice overhead. In most physician-owned practices, compensation is simply a result of the

A fixed expense is one that remains constant in total despite fluctuations in activity.

A variable expense is one that is uniform per unit but fluctuates in total in direct proportion to change in volume.

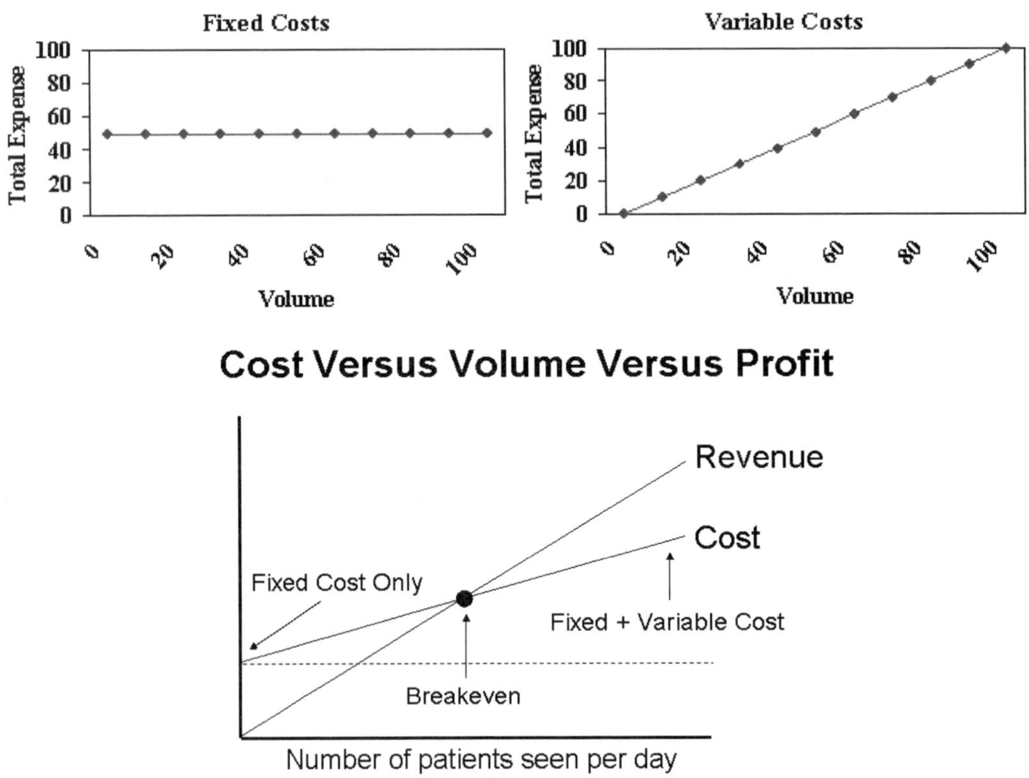

FIGURE 1-3 Expenses and Fixed/Variable Costs

monies left over after payment of all expenses. Most compensation plans include an incentive component. Therefore, the total paid to the physicians, ie, a combination of base pay, incentive pay, and benefits, should be reviewed.

The review process should use similar criteria for comparisons, such as industry standards by specialty and past operating results. Although industry standards and benchmarks are, in general, a good rule for guidance, in the final analysis, the individual practice and its performance relative to the monies left over for the employed and owner physicians count the most.

Salaries of employed physicians are a significant factor when a practice is for sale; they are considered during negotiations of the sale and in the determination of the new owner's practice operations. Excessive compensation may raise a red flag to prospective purchasers, though knowledgeable purchasers will compare productivity in both charges and wRVUs against industry benchmarks to determine the viability of physician compensation. The independent valuator who is knowledgeable in the methodologies of physician compensation in medical practices as well as medical practice operations should consider what is an appropriate compensation total. This figure should then be part of the calculations, depending on the methodology used. (Note: The income approach using a discounted cash flow methodology entails a *moving valuation*. This basically means that as the assumptions of physician compensation post-sale or employment initiation change, the valuation reflects this effect. In addition, in most instances nowadays, with hospital acquisitions, the sale entails greater emphasis on physician compensation maximization, effectively eliminating any value other than the tangible asset and possibly a *creation value* of the medical records.)

Enhanced Quality. The concepts of ACOs and PCMHs, as previously discussed, will be a major part of the landscape going forward. Therefore, the practice that can demonstrate quality performance and outcomes will likely receive more payment from Medicare; most probably, additional private payers will soon follow. Pilot programs are already underway to affect such forms of payment, yet fee-for-service will undoubtedly remain a part of the overall structure.

Discussions of quality in medicine are not new; providers have always emphasized this area among themselves. However, the big differential is that previously very little payment has been directly tied to quality indicators. One such system has been developed by Medicare. Originally called the Physician Quality Reporting Index (PQRI), it is now referred to as the Physician Quality Reporting System (PQRS). Here, a small portion of the total Medicare charges that a practice has generated within a year are available for additional payment, provided the practice can demonstrate and validate that it has met those requirements. While a good start, PQRI/PQRS has not dedicated sufficient monies within the overall payment structure to adequately provide an incentive to physicians and other providers to emphasize this area. Therefore, participation has been limited. Most physicians are very focused on high quality, regardless of the impact of payment. Nonetheless, the emphasis in payment now is more on enhanced quality outcomes, which may be achieved through the ACO and PCMH concepts.

The practice being prepared for sale must also be responsive now to documentation and demonstrations of quality. This capability is achieved best through a clinically integrated system, which, once again, is driving the consolidation of hospitals and physicians.

ACO Development. The ACO appears to be the vehicle of the future relative to the demonstration of the continuum of care and quality indicators. For most physician groups, forming their own ACO will be quite difficult. While there may be opportunities for larger multispecialty and some single-specialty groups to form an ACO, the likelihood of this occurring without the partnership of a health system or hospital, or a continuum of hospitals, will be challenging. Physicians, therefore, should consider their entire ACO strategy in the context of their physician/hospital alignment strategy, which may lead them to conclude that a sale of their practice is best. Ideally, physicians will play a prominent role in ACO leadership to achieve the ACO's essential goal of highest quality care at lowest possible cost.

Marketing Strategies for Selling

Once the decision has been made to sell the practice, strategies for completing the sale should be implemented. An important step is to secure qualified professional marketing assistance. This input will provide a clear understanding of the practice's value and marketability. Although the market has dwindled to a situation in which most interested purchasers are health systems or hospitals, having such a strategy is still appropriate.

Identifying Prospective Purchasers

Prospective buyers must be identified before market strategies can be put in place. Prospects are most likely to fall into the following categories:

- Other physicians
- Health systems/hospitals
- Health maintenance organizations
- Private corporations and venture capitalists

Health systems, both tertiary and primary or secondary care medical centers, and large medical practices are the most prominent purchasers. With accountable care and health care reform legislation at hand, practices are being acquired at a phenomenal pace, to the extent that many medical centers now own and employ hundreds of physicians and other providers. Indeed, these institutions are the primary "market" for purchase of practices.

As discussed, clearly, consolidation of providers is becoming the norm (ie, the emphasis toward quality and cost containment and payment is tied to the same through the PCMH/ACO structures) and is the greatest reason for practices being sold and physicians becoming employed or otherwise fully aligned with health systems or hospitals.

The vast majority of practice sales falls into this context. In addition, many practices are consolidating to increase their bargaining power with increasingly concentrated managed care organizations.

Thus, some practices will be sold and/or merged with other practices, which needs to be considered in the marketing process. Marketing to other physicians will be the best approach, factoring in a combination of perceived need and an ability to grow market share for the acquiring practice.

Outside Investors, Insurance Companies, and HMOs

Although they are very different entities, outside investors, insurance companies, and HMOs are grouped here for purposes of this discussion. There still may be some opportunity for the practice to be sold to one of these types of entities. Although becoming more rare (with health systems/hospitals being the primary purchasers of practices today), there still may be opportunities for the sale of the practice to private investors. This opportunity would primarily pertain to highly subspecialized entities that often have ancillary services as their primary product line. For example, a sleep center and sleep specialist physician may be more interested in selling to a for-profit entity. A gastroenterologist, for instance, may be more interested in selling to a private endoscopy company that would manage and own the practice and the corresponding endoscopy center. In these instances, there could well be a market in the private sector; therefore, private practicing physicians in such subspecialties should explore those possibilities.

Insurance companies may become purchasers of practices, particularly if they are part of a staff model HMO. The HMO is usually an independent, not-for-profit entity that can acquire practices and employ physicians in this setting. In some instances, the HMO may even partner with a health system or hospital and develop an employed physician network in such a consortium.

Private Practicing Physicians

Physicians still have an available market to sell to private practices. Although diminishing, the sale often takes the form of a merger of practices, wherein physicians grow through adding to an existing core practice or by their potential to create a new entity that houses the merged group. Although this chapter does not emphasize physician practice mergers as much as hospital and health systems acquisitions, mergers are a viable possibility.

As changes in reimbursement continue to force consolidation among hospitals and physicians, and managed care organizations become more inflexible in price negotiations, the strategy behind selling to a private practice (or even merging private practices) becomes much more challenging. However, the reason for this is that merging private practices does not always address the decreasing reimbursement issue. For example, hospitals receive higher payments from Medicare when billing as provider-based entities. Moreover, if hospitals bill for ancillary services as a hospital outpatient department, they also receive significantly higher reimbursement for the same services than a private entity. A merger might serve as an initial action before the ultimate step of becoming a part of a health system. Merging private entities does realize some additional influence with private payers, but does nothing for the additional payments hospitals receive from Medicare.

Becoming a part of a larger practice (or merging existing practices) is still a possibility for private practicing physicians preparing a practice for sale. The strategies discussed still apply in such situations. One major exception is that the compensation plan post-transaction in a private practice setting is often different. The private practicing group still has to manage its costs. There are no subsidies for compensating the physicians, as some hospitals will still do for their physicians post-transaction.

Private practicing physicians will still exist in the future, although they will have to develop a strategy on how to work within the changing payment paradigm, vis-à-vis, ACOs, PCMHs, bundled payments, and others. From a strategic view, selling the practice to a private entity or merging into or with another practice or practices must be considered in the context of a long-term viable strategy. Many large or mega groups have formed and are able to function almost as effectively as hospitals. By this, we mean that they have the financial and administrative capital to assure state-of-the-art processes, equipment, information technology, and overall management, much as hospitals invest today in large employed physician networks.

This option takes on a whole different strategy for selling physicians, as once again, the practice being sold is enveloped into a much larger system—much like it would be if it were purchased by a hospital. Such larger entities have developed to the level of sophistication necessary to compete with hospitals in this regard. The strategy and situation post-transaction may not be very different in terms of the adjustment and transitioning than it would be if it were sold to a hospital. Therefore, whether this is the best strategy must still be entertained.

Consultants and Attorneys

In the past, medical practices have used an independent broker agent to represent them in the sale of their practice. Although this is still done, on occasion the structure of the sales has become more complex than a simple broker agent can accomplish. Therefore, an independent consultant, along with a competent health care attorney, should make up the primary team to represent the practice in its sale.

Typically, a broker will charge on a percentage basis, yet the structure often lacks the professionalism required to complete such a transaction. However, a broker may still be the best option when a practice is only marketed to non-health system/hospital entities (ie, other physicians, private investors, etc).

The evolution of medical practice sales originally spawned a new industry several years ago, practice sale representation. Once a value has been placed on the practice, the consultant acts as the expert facilitator and negotiator to the selling physician. While individuals who represent the practice in its sale (somewhat as a broker) still exist, their duties have been largely transferred to highly competent health care experts, including consultants and attorneys. The consultants now complete the valuation work; review it and offer validation; develop and offer term sheets; and negotiate the transaction with the purchaser (usually a hospital). Specialized health care attorneys also play an active role in this process.

The health care consultant will usually provide the following consultative assistance:

- Advising the seller on the structuring of the sale
- Reviewing alternatives and options
- Completing and/or reviewing the practice valuation
- Identifying a buyer for the practice
- Leading negotiations
- Completing financial analyses and pro forma statements
- Reviewing and negotiating governance structure, post-transaction
- Establishing and negotiating the compensation terms and conditions
- Working with independent valuators of the practice, attorneys, and the purchaser's consultants/attorneys to expedite the transaction

Another possibility would be the use of an investment banking firm. While historically these transactions have not been large enough monetarily, some are now fitting into the mid-market transactional range ($10 million to $100 million, roughly) that many investment banking firms represent. Often, such deals include real estate, which easily places the total transactional value within the investment banker's purview. Investment bankers should be licensed to complete such transactions and typically will only deal in mid-sized to larger market agreements.

A sample consultant letter of agreement is presented in Figure 1-4.

Set forth below is the basis upon which Consultant will furnish services to Client:

John Doe, M.D. ("Dr. Doe," and/or the "Physician") herein contracts with Consultant ("Consultant") to provide consultative services pertaining to the negotiations that Dr. Doe's multi-specialty practice, DEF Practice ("DEF") is conducting with the local hospital in CITY (the "Hospital"). Prospectively, DEF (and possibly Dr. Doe) consummates the sale of the Practice and subsequent employment of Dr. Doe by the Hospital.

The work that Consultant will complete will be dependent upon the directives of the Physician in the course of the deliberations and negotiations. That work could entail behind the scenes review of defined structural, financial, and operational relationships with the development or review of applicable documentation, memorializing the agreed-upon terms and conditions. While this agreement (the "Agreement") does not specifically entail drafting of applicable agreements, if requested, a separate agreement will be completed wherein Consultant would assist the Physician accordingly.

This Agreement documents Consultant's work in the context of what is anticipated to be completed on behalf of the Physician in this situation. Consultant will not negotiate directly with the Hospital regarding the specific terms and conditions and economic ramifications of the Physician providing professional services to the Hospital in such a setting. Further, Consultant will not communicate with representatives of DEF unless requested by Dr. Doe to do so. Rather, our function will be to review and analyze the proposed terms and conditions and provide expert consultation to Dr. Doe as he processes the offer and overall go-forward structure of working for the Hospital. This will allow him to thoroughly and effectively evaluate his alternatives and decide accordingly.

Consultant's fees for this Assignment are estimated to not exceed $_______, assuming normal processes occur (this does not include work beyond that defined herein). If additional time and resultant fees are required, Consultant will obtain approval from Dr. Doe and memorialize the authorization via an additional written agreement.

Professional fees will be billed to the Physician on an hourly basis (in quarter hour increments). While no on-site time is anticipated, if this is authorized, an additional agreement would be required to expand the fee structure. The professional fees will be billed at the end of each calendar month and paid within ten days of the billing date.

FIGURE 1-4 Sample Consulting Letter of Agreement

In addition, the Physician agrees to reimburse Consultant's out-of-pocket expenses incurred to complete this assignment (at this time Consultant does not anticipate any significant reimbursable expenses as travel on-site is not planned). Nonetheless, Consultant will provide documentation of any out-of-pocket expenses incurred and billed. Payment will be due within ten days of invoice date.

Should the Physician request additional work from Consultant after the completion of these initiatives, a separate agreement will be developed at that time.

Indemnification by the Physician

The Physician will indemnify and hold harmless Consultant, its members, shareholders, employees, independent contractors, agents, and other personnel from and against any and all claims, demands, liabilities, losses, damages, costs, and expenses (including reasonable attorney's fees, court costs, and other expenses incurred in defending against claims or otherwise connected therewith) (hereinafter a "Loss" or "Losses") resulting in any manner, directly or indirectly, from the gross negligence or intentional acts or omissions of the Physician, its members, directors, officers, employees, independent contractors, or agents.

Apart from our independent investigation, Consultant will have to rely in part on the information provided by the Physician. To that extent the Physician will indemnify and hold harmless Consultant and its personnel from and against any claims, liabilities, costs, and expenses (including, without limitation, attorneys' fees and the time of Consultant personnel involved) brought against, paid, or incurred by Consultant at any time and in any way arising out of or relating to the information provided by the Physician and relied upon by Consultant, except to the extent finally determined to have resulted from the gross negligence, professional malpractice, willful or intentional misconduct acts or omissions of Consultant personnel. This provision shall survive the termination of this agreement for any reason.

Indemnification by Consultant

Consultant will indemnify and hold harmless the Physician, its members, shareholders, employees, independent contractors, agents, and other personnel from and against any and all claims, demands, liabilities, losses, damages, costs, and expenses (including reasonable attorney fees, court costs, and other expenses incurred in defending against claims or

FIGURE 1-4 Sample Consulting Letter of Agreement (*continued*)

otherwise connected therewith) (hereinafter a "Loss" or "Losses") resulting in any manner, directly or indirectly, from the gross negligence, professional malpractice, or intentional acts or omissions of Consultant, its members, shareholders, employees, independent contractors, or agents.

Consultant's Privacy Policy

Attached via Exhibit I is Consultant's Privacy Policy.

Consultant's Confidentiality and Non-Disclosure Agreement

Attached via Exhibit II is Consultant's Confidentiality and Non-Disclosure Agreement.

____________________________ ____________

John Doe, M.D. Date

For Consultant:

____________________________ ____________

Date

FIGURE 1-4 Sample Consulting Letter of Agreement (*continued*)

Exhibit I
Consultant
Privacy Policy

Our Commitment to the Privacy of Your Information

We are dedicated to protecting the privacy of your identifiable information, including any identifiable protected health information that you may disclose to us. We value your trust and we want you to understand what types of information we collect, how we use that information, and the steps we take to protect individually identifiable patient health information (or "patient health information"). We will treat patient health information that you disclose to us with respect and in accordance with this Privacy Policy and applicable law.

Our Privacy Policy

We will provide all of our clients with a copy of our current Privacy Policy on an annual basis.

We may revise our Privacy Policy from time to time. If we revise our Privacy Policy, we will provide a copy of the new Privacy Policy to you.

You are welcome to contact us at any time to discuss our privacy policies.

We will maintain physical, electronic, and procedural safeguards to protect patient health information we obtain from our clients.

We will not sell patient health information.

We will not share patient health information with third parties, except as permitted by law and as described in this Privacy Policy.

We will require our subcontractors and agents to whom we disclose patient health information to adhere to our Privacy Policy standards.

Please read on for details about our privacy practices. Our Privacy Policy includes examples of the types of information we may collect and the kinds of entities with whom we may share information. These examples are illustrative and should not be considered a complete inventory of our information collection, use, and disclosure practices.

Information We May Collect

We may obtain information to provide you with products and/or services you have requested and to service your needs. Examples of the types of patient health information we may collect, and the uses to which we may put that information, include:

- Patient medical records, including paper and electronic records, in the process of performing chart audits
- Patient insurance and billing information, including Explanation of Benefits, patient diagnosis and procedure information, and financial status of the patient's bill as it relates to billing reviews
- Patient charts, records, names, and personally identifiable health information that may be inadvertently encountered in the course of conducting other services we provide such as:
    - Operational assessments
    - Physician and staff education sessions
    - Marketing and strategic planning

How Your Information May Be Used and Disclosed by Us

We may disclose your identifiable information, including patient health information, in the following types of situations:

Disclosures to Service Providers

We may disclose the information we collect, including patient health information, to individuals and companies that provide services on your behalf. Such individuals and organizations may be:

- Assisting you (or us) with a project for you
- Providing services to you or on your behalf, including administrative services and customer assistance
- Preparing, printing, copying, and delivering statements and other documents
- Third-party billing companies
- Application service providers

Uses and Disclosures Permitted by Law

We may use and disclose your information, including your patient health information, for our internal purposes (such as for our proper management and administration) and to carry out our present and future legal responsibilities—but only if such uses and disclosures are permitted under applicable confidentiality laws. We also may use and disclose your information, including your patient health information, as otherwise permitted or required by law.

We may use and disclose your information—but not your patient health information—to market products and services to you, or to permit third parties to market products and services to you. You may request in writing that we not use your information to market products or services to you.

No Uses or Disclosures of Patient Health Information for Other Purposes

We will not share any patient health information we collect with third parties, except as described in our Privacy Policy. We will not use or disclose your patient health information for purposes of marketing our goods or services. Also, we will not disclose your patient health information to any third party for any marketing purposes, unless expressly permitted by you and applicable law. We will never sell patient health information.

We may de-identify your information, including your patient health information, and use and disclose such de-identified information for any purpose. Any patient health information we de-identify will be de-identified in accordance with the current Standards for Privacy of Individually Identifiable Health Information promulgated by the U.S. Department of Health and Human Services pursuant to the Health Insurance Portability and Accountability Act of 1996.

Our Security Procedures

We maintain procedures and technology designed to prevent unauthorized access to your information, including patient health information. We maintain physical, electronic, and procedural protections in accordance with applicable standards to protect patient health information. We restrict access to patient health information to our employees, our subcontractors and agents, your service providers for legitimate business purposes to assist in providing products and services to you. Our employees, subcontractors, and agents are subject to disciplinary action for violations of our Privacy Policy.

Exhibit II
Consultant
Confidentiality and Non-Disclosure Agreement

This Confidentiality and Non-Disclosure Agreement (the "Agreement") is entered into and made effective as of this ________ day of Month, Year (the "Effective Date"), by and between John Doe, M.D., (the "Physician") and Consultant ("Consultant"), with respect to the considerable secret, confidential, and proprietary information, intellectual property rights, and know-how which the Physician owns, and which the Physician will or might provide to Consultant, or Consultant might otherwise become aware of during its engagement.

In consideration of the mutual promises and covenants made herein, the Physician and Consultant agree as follows:

(a) Consultant agrees that all information, whether or not in writing, of a private, secret, or confidential nature concerning the Physician's business, business relationships, or financial affairs (collectively, "Proprietary Information") is and shall be the exclusive property of the Physician. By way of illustration, but not limitation, Proprietary Information may include inventions, products, processes, methods, techniques, formulas, compositions, compounds, projects, developments, plans, research data, clinical data, financial data, personnel data, computer programs, source code and programming information, customer and supplier lists, and contacts at or knowledge of customers or prospective customers of the Physician, whether in written, electronic, oral, or any other form. Consultant will not disclose any Proprietary Information to any person or entity other than its employees who have a need to know about such information in order to render services to the Physician or use the same for any purposes (other than in the performance of its duties as a Consultant to the Physician) without written approval by an officer of the Physician, either during or after its engagement with the Physician, unless and until such Proprietary Information has become public knowledge without fault by Consultant.

(b) Consultant agrees that all files, letters, memoranda, reports, records, data, sketches, drawings, laboratory notebooks, program listings, or other written, photographic, or other tangible material containing Proprietary Information, whether created by Consultant or its employees or provided by the Physician, which shall come into its custody or possession, shall be and are the exclusive property of the Physician to be used by Consultant only in the performance of its services for the Physician. All such materials or copies thereof and all tangible property of the Physician in the custody or possession of Consultant shall be delivered to the Physician, upon the later of (i) a request by the Physician or (ii) termination of its engagement. After such delivery, Consultant may retain any such materials or copies thereof or any such tangible property.

(c) Consultant agrees that its obligation not to disclose or to use information and materials of the types set forth in paragraphs (a) and (b) above and its obligation to return materials and tangible property, set forth in paragraph (b) above, also extends to such types of information, materials, and tangible property of customers of the Physician or suppliers to the Physician or other third parties who may have disclosed or entrusted the same to the Physician or to Consultant.

(d) Nothing in this Agreement shall be deemed to affect Consultant's existing ownership rights in its existing inventions, software, or other intellectual property.

(e) In the event that Consultant is requested or required by subpoena or other court order to disclose any Proprietary Information, Consultant will provide immediate notice of such request to the Physician and will use reasonable efforts to resist disclosure, until an appropriate protective order may be sought, or a waiver of compliance with the provisions of this Agreement granted. If, in the absence of a protective order or the receipt of a waiver hereunder, Consultant is nonetheless, in the written opinion of its counsel, legally required to disclose Proprietary Information, then, in such event, Consultant may disclose such information without liability hereunder, provided that the Physician has been given a reasonable opportunity to review the text of such disclosure before it is made and that the disclosure is limited to only the Proprietary Information specifically required to be disclosed.

1. Warranties and Representations

Consultant warrants and represents that its performance of all the terms of this Agreement and as Consultant of the Physician does not and will not breach any agreement to keep in confidence proprietary information, knowledge, or data acquired by Consultant in confidence or in trust prior to its engagement with the Physician, and that Consultant will not disclose to the Physician or induce the Physician to use any confidential or proprietary information or material previously acquired and belonging to any previous employer or others.

2. Miscellaneous

The invalidity or unenforceability of any provision of this Agreement shall not affect the validity or enforceability of any other provision of this Agreement.

(a) This Agreement supersedes all prior agreements, written or oral, between Consultant and the Physician relating to the subject matter of this Agreement.

(b) This Agreement shall be binding upon Consultant's successors, subsidiaries, affiliates, or assigns and upon Consultant's directors, officers, employees, partners, representatives, and agents of any kind. This Agreement shall inure to the benefit of the Physician and its successors and assigns.

(c) No delay or omission by the Physician in exercising any right under this Agreement will operate as a waiver of that or any other right. A waiver or consent given by the Physician on any one occasion is effective only in that instance and will not be construed as a bar to or waiver of any right on any other occasion.

(d) Consultant expressly consents to be bound by the provisions of this Agreement for the benefit of the Physician or any successor, subsidiary, or affiliate thereof to which Consultant might provide services without the necessity that this Agreement be re-signed at the time of such transfer.

(e) The restrictions contained in this Agreement are necessary for the protection of the business and goodwill of the Physician and are considered by Consultant to be reasonable for such purpose. Consultant agrees that any breach of this Agreement is likely to cause the Physician substantial and irreparable damage and therefore, in the event of any such breach, Consultant agrees that the Physician, in addition to such other remedies as may be available at law or in equity, shall be entitled to specific performance and other injunctive relief. Should litigation or an alternative dispute resolution mechanism be instituted to enforce any provision of this Agreement, the prevailing party shall be entitled to recover all costs, including reasonable attorney's fees.

(f) The parties consent to the jurisdiction of the State of ________ for any lawsuit that arises from a dispute of any nature among the parties.

(g) This Agreement expires one (1) year from the date of the last disclosure under this Agreement.

Consultant and the Physician acknowledge that both parties have carefully read this Agreement and understand and agree to all of the provisions in this Agreement.

Date: ________________________________

Consultant

Date: ________________________________

John Doe, M.D.

Other Ways to Purchase or Sell a Practice

A medical practice can also be sold through more traditional methods, such as networking and advertising. While it is not essential to use a professional consultant, it is usually best to do so. However, if the decision is to complete this process without outside assistance, several approaches may be used together to find a viable buyer. After identifying a prospective buyer (usually a hospital), it will still be best to turn over the facilitation and negotiations to an experienced consultant and/or attorney.

Networking

Networking is one of the best ways to notify others that the practice is for sale. Inform various contacts, such as medical supply sales associates, pharmaceutical representatives, and hospital administrators, of your decision to gain exposure to other health care professionals. The American Medical Association's physician placement service provides the names of physicians who are seeking positions. Other sources include bulletin boards in hospitals and graduate schools. Speak with college placement directors. Consider using direct mail as a means to sell the practice. Review specialty or association journal advertisements to gain insight into what practices are for sale and their locations. In summary, with these mediums considered, hospitals (essentially those in which physicians have practiced during their private practice tenure) are still the most likely viable purchaser.

Advertising

If you choose to advertise, make sure your advertisement is credible and does not sound too good to be true. Include ample information but not too much. Describe the type of practice (specialty), approximate earnings, general location (regional area), and specify rural or urban setting. Listing the sales price of the practice is not always advisable, yet this may be appropriate in some markets or when you want to sell quickly. Once the advertisement is placed, keep a record of the responses. Document every telephone call received or made, noting all information you obtain from prospective purchasers. Figure 1-5

G.P. Practice
Modern 4 operatory practice
$525,000 income. Profitable.
Midland, Michigan, area
(telephone number)

FIGURE 1-5 Advertisement

is an example of an effective advertisement. Be careful about putting offers or acceptances in writing (or verbally) without the advice of an attorney.

Professional Assistance

Selling a medical practice is no small undertaking. The seller should realize the value of the practice and not be reluctant to obtain professional assistance including a qualified independent appraiser or valuator. Competent legal and financial advice from brokers, consultants, accountants, and attorneys, if used properly, also play a vital role in the outcome of the sale, rendering substantial dividends. In addition to the earlier discussion regarding expert consultants, the following section further explores the use and value of attorneys, accountants, and possibly even brokers (although the need for brokers has lessened dramatically in that little monies are paid up front unless a great amount of real estate and tangible assets are included).

The Attorney

The primary function of the attorney is to help document (and sometimes negotiate) legal matters, interpret the law, and draft and finalize agreements. The attorney also protects physicians from regulatory and legal pitfalls, including Stark law provisions, anti-kickback statues, and state regulations. Engage a competent attorney with experience in drafting physician employment contracts, leases, asset or stock purchase agreements, and bills of conveyance and partnership agreements. If the medical practice is a corporation, the attorney should have a working knowledge of corporate law. Also, the attorney must be familiar with business documentation through directors' and stockholders' meetings and the minutes of those meetings. Above all, the attorney should be extremely knowledgeable of health care law, and not just a generalist.

The Accountant

Before agreeing to a sales contract, seek the advice of an accountant on tax matters such as allocation of assets, compensation, personnel policies, and installment sale treatment. Find an accountant who has experience working with physicians and is familiar with medical practice operations (or similar professional practices, such as attorneys and dentists). An attorney and an accountant are in the best positions to advise on taxes. (Note: Most practice sales are of the "assets," not the legal entity. This is done to avert liability on unknowns and/or contingencies of the legal entity [usually a corporate or limited liability company]. As such, these transactions carry specific tax ramifications [both sales taxes in some states and federal/state income/franchise taxes] that call for expertise of this nature. Intangible asset value or goodwill is a rare occurrence nowadays, so this area of tax consideration is not applicable. Even so, there are other areas of opportunity for legitimate tax savings within the existing structures currently being completed.)

The Broker

The need for brokers is diminishing, given that many purchasers of practices are health systems and hospitals. However, if the practice is for sale to private entities, usually other physicians, and there is a need to market it, the broker serves as agent, or matchmaker. The broker acts for the selling physician after the value of the practice has been placed. Ideally, the broker has knowledge of prospective buyers and will ultimately bring the buyer and seller together.

The Consultant

As discussed, health care consultants are becoming more prevalent in response to the increasing complexities of the health care industry. Consultants could include accountants and lawyers but more often are experienced, specialized experts that assist physicians, hospitals, and other health care providers with integration. Examine the experience and reputation of this individual or firm. Some firms can provide appraisal, accounting, and tax analysis; legal expertise; and the experience needed to negotiate the agreement. Other firms may specialize in only one or two areas. Although using one firm may be a convenient option, it may be more appropriate to involve different professionals, because you receive different levels of opinion, understanding, and expertise. However, if the practice is being sold to a health system or hospital, the consultant should handle all but perhaps the final definitive agreements that the attorney reviews and drafts.

For either scenario, select a consultant with these characteristics:

- Reputation for accurate work
- Experience doing the work well, including financial analyses, valuations, and negotiation skills
- Good references and credentials supporting work, technical ability, market knowledge, and understanding of the scope of the transaction

Qualified, competent, and expert consultants will prevent you from losing both money and your reputation. Preferably, this firm should be one that also represents health systems, as their consultants not only will know and understand the operations of a hospital-employed physician network, but also they will know how hospitals "think" in such transactions. Obviously, consultants are not able to represent both the hospital and the practice within the same transaction. What we mean is that the most valuable consultants to assist and represent the practice would be ones who also have experience representing hospitals. This experience will help immensely with expediting the transaction and the economic outcomes of the deal (ie, maximizing value or compensation).

Governance

Governance makes up a major part of any transaction post-sale. This is especially the case when physicians are merging a practice with another practice, but even more so now when physicians are selling to health systems or hospitals. While the paradigm of such transactions in the 1990s (and even the early part of the 2000s) was rarely considered, nowadays, when physicians are selling their practices to health systems or hospitals, governance is one of the major topics—almost as important as the economics itself.

Various governance structures have been established. These typically make up the discussion (and ultimately the agreements) relative to day-to-day operational decisions, through major transactional decisions, and even in many cases, to a management role within the hospital's service line. For example, there have been numerous cardiology transactions in recent years, largely driven by the fact that reimbursement for diagnostic testing (such as nuclear studies and echocardiograms) has been reduced dramatically by Medicare. To date, hospitals have not experienced such reductions. Therefore, while hospitals cannot compensate the physician directly for the increased reimbursement they realize from acquiring the ancillary services, overall the transaction can be structured in such a way to create a better economic outcome for the physician. However, many of the cardiologists that are selling their practices to hospitals (usually for no upfront money—only the tangible asset value, as such) are very concerned about governance, and therefore are placing high levels of importance in the negotiation process concerning this matter.

In many cases, governance becomes more of a dyadic management model wherein the physicians work almost in a partnership role with the hospital to make governance decisions. Moreover, in some cases these structures are set up whereby the physicians (again, using cardiologists as an example) will help the hospital manage the entire service line, which would include not only the ambulatory practice, but also the diagnostic testing, rehabilitation, and perhaps even assistance in managing the inpatient side of the hospital's services.

Thus, governance must be a major consideration within any sale, especially when physicians are going to continue long-term employment post-transaction. Hospital medical staff by-laws and similar documents should be obtained and reviewed. This process applies to private sales (ie, to other physicians and investors) and especially to hospital acquisitions.

Unwind Provisions

Every transaction needs to have documented understandings and agreements relative to the unwind provisions. While most (if not all) transactions should be viewed as long-term and enduring, this is not always the case. Therefore, the unwind provisions must be outlined and agreed upon. They should be regarded almost like a prenuptial agreement in the event that a "marriage" does not work.

Unwind provisions are varied, but usually will allow for some protection of both parties. For example, for selling physicians, the provisions should at least protect the physicians' return to a private practice setting, as long as no direct competition is created for the acquiring practice or health system. It is more difficult to justify this same provision for a private practice that is unwinding another private practice physician, allowing that individual to go back into private practice. However, that physician should have the ability to continue earning a living within the area that the practice had been developed. Needless to say, this matter is negotiable.

As relates to hospitals and restrictive covenants or non-competition restrictions (in essence, what we are referring to in the example), the key point is to not create a competitive situation that benefits other direct competitors of the hospitals. Usually this applies to either a large group that may not be active at that hospital or another hospital or health system. "Non-compete" clauses are generally disfavored in the law and must be specific as to geography, scope, and time. State laws vary; in some states non-compete clauses are prohibited except in very narrow circumstances.

From the standpoint of the other unwind provisions, these are based on the agreed-upon considerations at that time. For example, selling physicians may be able to acquire the assets of the practice at the unwind. Most often, these terms would be established on a first right of refusal of that physician, plus the ability to buy the assets at the independently valued fair market value.

As for employees and other client leads (even non-patients who might be acquiring health care services from the practice for certain products and services), typically these would require some non-solicitation terms and agreements. Again, these terms would be negotiable, but often non-solicitation terms are required for the physician to go back into a private practice setting and be absolved from any violation of that right by not soliciting employees of the practice for a certain period of time (usually at least one year).

Thus, the unwind provisions should address these key points to a degree that few (if any) gray areas exist.

Chapter 2 on disengagement provides additional information on practice unwinds.

Dissolution

Once you have a contract for the sale of the practice, that business entity will eventually be dissolved. Many components of a dissolution must be addressed to ensure that the seller does not lose money. As mentioned, most sellers are selling only specific medical practice assets, not the entire entity. Generally, they do not include certain items that the buyer is not interested in purchasing. For example, most cash and related items are not included in the purchase. Accounts receivable are usually not included, and assets such as automobiles, miscellaneous deposits, and some prepaid items are seldom part of the transaction. These items must be disposed of or distributed before the legal entity housing the practice is formally dissolved, even if the physician continues on as an employee.

In this section, several of these items are discussed, and ways to dissolve the remainder of the practice while maximizing the income from these efforts are recommended.

Cash Equivalents, and Other Assets

All cash and bank accounts should be distributed to the owners before the sale of the practice, assuming that they are selling the practice assets and not the whole entity. Bank accounts should be reconciled, with any remaining money distributed to the owners. Other assets not specifically included in the sale should also be transferred to the proper individual. For example, an automobile once owned by the practice (whether the practice is a corporation, partnership, or sole proprietorship) should be transferred to the individual who will assume its private ownership. Old equipment that is not being purchased by the buyer must be disposed of. If it cannot be relocated easily or if it does not have appreciable market value, it can be donated, for example, to a developing country. Contact your specialty society for information on making these types of arrangements.

If the buyer does not want to purchase all the furniture and office equipment, what will you do with it? How much will you have to pay to move it? Where will you store it? Or how will you dispose of it? Consider contacting used furniture sellers for a modest redemption value or donate items to reputable charities.

Accounts Receivable

In a practice acquisition, patients are a vital part of the sales transaction; however, the accounts receivable are usually not purchased. Therefore, the seller should have mechanisms in place to collect all outstanding balances. In this way, the total earnings from the sale can be increased, because accounts receivable are not usually calculated in the actual valuation. (Note: This matter is negotiable, but usually hospitals do not want to purchase the accounts receivable. They will, however, allow them to be collected by their newly employed staff [for a market-based collection fee]). Collection of outstanding balances brings additional revenue to the selling physicians; the more that can be collected from outstanding accounts, the more monies the former owners receive. It is preferable for collections to continue under the former practice name and billing protocols.

Even when accounts receivable are not included in the assets purchased, new owners may agree to bill and collect outstanding receivables as of the sale date. Collections are easier for new owners because they are equipped and responsible for collecting their own new receivables, and the former owners benefit by not having to be directly involved. Typically, the collection arrangement is based on a percentage of collection.

Collection of all accounts receivable should take place during the first 60 days after the sale. Once patients learn physicians have sold a practice, particularly if the former owners/physicians are leaving, collecting becomes more difficult. An aggressive collections approach may be needed to ensure that most outstanding receivables are collected.

Accounts Payable

As the dissolution proceeds, the new physicians/owners should assume responsibility for all outstanding obligations. Separating all liabilities incurred before the sale's closing date is important. If purchasers are acquiring selected assets of the entity (as opposed to the entire entity), in most instances the accounts payable remain the obligation of the previous owners. In the interest of both parties, list the accounts payable by vendor on an exhibit to the purchase agreement or attached as a memorandum to avoid discrepancies. Sellers should use the proceeds from the sale of the practice plus the collected accounts receivable to pay them off promptly. It is not in the best interest of selling physicians or acquiring purchasers to have lingering accounts payable that may cause a negative reflection on either.

The purchase agreement should address any carryover of liabilities; these are obligations unknown as of the date of closing, but pertain to events occurring prior to the closing and are the responsibility of the previous owners. To illustrate, office supplies are received in inventory five days before the practice sale is closed; the new owners include these supplies in the purchase price. If an invoice for these supplies comes after the sale, the selling physicians are responsible for paying the invoice.

Contingent liabilities, such as outstanding claims and lawsuits, are the obligation of the former owners and are usually addressed in the purchase agreement. The new purchasers are not subject to these claims, especially if the transaction is an asset purchase (as opposed to a legal entity purchase). No consideration is necessary as sellers plan and manage the dissolution of ownership.

Tax Considerations

Tax considerations are paramount in the overall dissolution of the medical practice. A qualified tax accountant can advise on and assist with these matters. This information assures the sellers of both proper treatment of income for tax purposes and optimum tax savings. The sellers of the practice must consider many tax implications. Following is a review of these implications.

Property Taxes

Typically, taxes on property are assessed annually; the payment date varies, depending on local authorities. Property taxes are assessed at local (ie, city and county) levels. Also, some states assess property, including property other than real estate, for taxation. If property taxes are prepaid, tax liability should be prorated for fair allocation for the remainder of the period. The seller's share is based on the portion of the assessed period that the practice was owned. Likewise, the buyers' amount to be paid is easily determined using the tax assessment date and the period for which they were paid. Occasionally, property taxes are assessed in arrears, ie, they are billed for the year that has just ended, even if it is after the date the practice closed. These taxes can be estimated and prorated as of the closing. An alternative is to assess prior owners for a portion of the year's taxes when the tax bill is received. If real estate is included in the transaction, the closing attorney will automatically prorate taxes, insurance, and all escrow accounts.

Payroll Taxes

Payroll taxes are the responsibility of practice owners. The prior owners' tax liability for persons employed by the practice extends to the time of the practice closing. The new owners assume that liability as of the date of acquisition, if the new owners continue to employ the staff. If the date of closing is in the middle of a pay period, payroll taxes must be prorated.

A clear separation of employment should be made. That is, employees should be officially terminated from the prior owners' employment and rehired by the new owners. Payroll tax payments are much less complicated, and it is better for personnel policies and benefit purposes, if this procedure is followed. It is particularly beneficial when practice assets are acquired as opposed to the entire entity. If the entire entity (ie, a corporation) is acquired, the employees are typically part of the transaction, and no official termination and rehire mechanisms are in place.

Sales Taxes/Local Taxes

Usually, sales and local taxes do not apply to these transactions. However, state and local authorities are becoming more aggressive in levying taxes on such transactions among professionals. Check your state, county, and local/city regulations to determine if any such taxes are applicable (or potentially applicable).

Income/Franchise Taxes

From the seller's perspective, as much of the sales price as feasible should be allocated to goodwill and other intangibles. The value of these assets is taxed as a capital gain, which currently is at a maximum rate of 28%. Further, an installment sale, if allowed, will make it possible to spread the tax liability over the installment period. Tangible assets, however, are treated differently. If the equipment has been mostly depreciated, anything received for it beyond the net book value will be taxed as ordinary income in the year of the sale. Ordinary income tax rates vary, depending on the legal structure of the entity. In addition, if there is a pass-through to the individual owner, that person's personal income tax rate will affect the income tax rates.

Income taxes are due at least quarterly, usually made through an estimated tax payment schedule. For example, if the practice is sold on April 30, the seller cannot delay the payment of any tax liability stemming from the sale until the end of the year. A quarterly estimate, which would be due after the end of the second quarter, would be required, based on the projected profit from the sale and resulting tax liability.

Legal Entity Termination

Once the practice has been sold, the legal entity (assuming that it was not sold) should be officially dissolved, whether it is a corporation, partnership, or limited liability company. Even a sole proprietorship should be dissolved, at least for local business licensing purposes. Dissolving legal entities is quite simple. Usually, the only requirement is registration with the secretary of state, documenting the date and time of the dissolution. When the final tax return is completed for the entity, the filer can check off the appropriate space on the form to note that it is the final return. Also adhere to these measures when meeting the local, state, and federal requirements.

The official dissolution process need not take place immediately following the sale of the practice. Selling physicians will need to follow up in many areas. Additionally, the legal entity should continue for some time (up to one year) after the closure to pay off final liabilities and collect remaining accounts receivable. Also, pension plan considerations include funding requirements and other responsibilities. This transitional period after the sale provides time to resolve lingering matters but should not create any additional liabilities or negative implications.

Refer to Chapter 6 for additional information on practice dissolution.

Transitioning to the New Owner

Most, if not all, of the considerations for transitioning that apply to purchasers also apply to sellers. These are discussed in the following section.

Patients

Think about the impact on your patients when you make the decision to sell. Patients see physicians as confidants and treat them with respect. It can be upsetting when physicians leave or join a practice or even when they become employed by a hospital or health system. (Note: Most hospitals downplay the fact that physicians are employed by them, although for Medicare and Medicaid billing purposes, they must claim the clinic and ancillaries as "hospital/outpatient based." This process allows hospitals opportunities to bill at higher rates under the Hospital Outpatient Perspective Payment System [HOPPS] and Hospital Outpatient Department [HOPD] and Provider Based Billing [PBB] rates.)

Patients deserve to receive information about staffing changes and an explanation of what effect it will have on them, if any. In some cases, state regulation including policies of the state medical licensure board may control the physicians' obligation to notify patients. Although networking makes it impossible to keep the sale confidential, patients need official notification when a change in medical practice ownership occurs. An exception exists when no changes are made in the physician staff (ie, when a hospital system purchases a practice). Again, it is actually preferable for the transition to be as seamless as possible. Although, if the community becomes aware of the sale, a letter of reassurance to all patients is vital. When a transition occurs due to retirement, announce it by a letter to the patients. Figure 1-6 is a sample letter announcing retirement.

[Letterhead]

Date:

An open letter to my patients:

With mixed emotions, I announce my impending retirement from practice.

I will, on the one hand, miss my patients and colleagues. On the other hand, I look forward to living a more relaxed life with my lovely spouse.

I feel certain that you will be in good hands with Dr.______ with whom I have worked closely for the past several months. If our office does not hear otherwise, I'll turn over your records to her. Dr.______ will be taking over my office and equipment when I depart. I envy her training; it's so much better today than when I was in school, and I'd be pleased if you confirmed my judgment of her by selecting her as your physician. I am very much impressed by the quality of her work and I think you might be also.

If for some reason you choose not to ask Dr.________ to care for your health needs, you should select another physician. If you will advise my office of your selection (in writing), not later than the end of the month, we will transfer your records to your new physician, or if regulations permit, provide them to you.

I will continue seeing patients at regular office hours until the end of this month. If you do not have an appointment between now and then and want to stop by, I'd be pleased to see you between 3 p.m. and 5 p.m. on Wednesday afternoons (when I am not seeing regularly scheduled patients). It's been a pleasure for me to have been of service to you.

Sincerely,

____

Dr. John Doe

FIGURE 1-6 Letter Announcing Retirement

Managed Care Organizations

Managed care contracts are not automatically transferred to new owners. Occasionally, managed care organizations approve the assignment of contracts; often they require a complete recredentialing process and assignment of new provider numbers. Determine the status of the managed care contracts prior to consummating the purchase agreement. Sellers should cooperate with prospective buyers to determine if the new owners can assume managed care contracts.

Personnel

Personnel issues likely entail the most work in practice transitions. When only practice assets are being purchased, consider terminating all employees (hospitals most assuredly will). The acquiring party can choose to rehire specific individuals. Retaining practice employees who know the patients will help curb patient defection in the ownership transition. Other personnel actions need to be considered and are discussed as follows.

Employee Hiring and Firing

Employee hiring and firing must be handled with extreme caution by buyers and sellers. From the sellers' perspective, each employee should be officially terminated. This action affects benefits such as termination pay, severance pay, accrued vacation, and accrued sick leave. These benefits must be reconciled between both parties and addressed with the employees. Not all benefits result in a liability to the sellers of the practice.

For example, assuming that sellers recognize accrued vacation as a liability, the sellers and buyers can negotiate this point for assumption of liability. If the buyers agree to recognize accrued vacation as time off during the first year of ownership, the two parties may resolve this circumstance accordingly. In contrast, buyers may not want to extend paid vacation leave, under the assumption that the employee has not earned that vacation under the new employment relationship. The terminated employee may warrant a cash payment by the sellers for the accrued vacation.

In addition, employees may be subject to state laws regarding notification of termination of their health insurance coverage and eligibility under the Consolidated Omnibus Budget Reconciliation Act (COBRA). These matters must be discussed, outlined, and resolved prior to the announcement of sale. Employees are entitled to clear communication of benefits.

Record Keeping

Record keeping and documentation of pay (eg, salaries, overtime, time off) must be maintained by sellers. If employees are officially terminated and rehired by the new entity, sellers are subject to wage and hour audits and other potential reviews involving personnel actions during their ownership of the practice.

Health Insurance Benefits

Health insurance benefits must be transferred to new owners. If the practice employs 20 or more people, the new owners are subject to a continuation of coverage under the provisions of the COBRA regulations. This process potentially entails an additional cost to the employees, as COBRA requires employees to pay the full premium for health insurance.

Other Benefits

Employer obligations related to unemployment benefits and workers' compensation should accrue to the sellers, and should be fully investigated and disclosed. Other benefits must be effectively transitioned from the old practice to the new. Sick leave, disability insurance, retirement benefits, and life insurance must be terminated or converted. When the practice is acquired, whether it consists of the actual legal entity or only its assets, the new owners will establish a new benefits package and are not required to offer or assume that of the prior owners'. Employees can benefit from the sale if the new owners offer an improved benefits package; this often occurs when physician owners sell to a larger health system (eg, a hospital, private corporation) with a comprehensive benefits plan.

Medical Records

If all medical records are transferred to the buyers, there should be a stipulation in the contract that allows the sellers access to records for at least 10 years beyond the last day a patient was treated, in the event litigation occurs. This time frame could be longer, depending on physician specialty and state law. The malpractice insurer for the practice retains comprehensive information on retention of medical records.

If maintenance or responsibility of all old medical records is not assumed by the buyers, the sellers must maintain and preserve the integrity of all records not transferred to another physician until the statute of limitations expires. In that situation, the sellers need to consider some of the following issues: Where will you store the records? What will it cost you? Should you add the cost of their maintenance to the selling price?

The Phase-Out Agreement

A phase-out agreement is a legal contract that defines how the buyers and sellers will operate during a specified period after the sale. This agreement must be decided before the sellers officially leave the practice. (Obviously, this agreement would not be applicable in any transactions wherein the seller is subsequently employed by the buyer, unless it occurs some time later when the physician leaves the practice.) It defines the transfer of all or part of the ownership during a specified period. Through this document, a phase-in buyer or phase-out seller is arranging for both parties to work together.

The phase-out agreement should do the following:

- Define how long the selling physician will remain in the practice.
- Define the duties of the buyer and seller. (Patient distribution and hours worked should be considered. It must be very clear that in case of disagreement, the new owners will prevail.)
- Establish a level of compensation (including fringe benefits).
- Establish the actual purchase price by conducting an independent valuation.
- Arrange for parties to exchange monies (at least in deposit form or as earnest money placed in escrow) prior to the official closing during the phase-out period.
- Enable the purchaser to assume more responsibility as time passes. (The purchasing physician cares for more patients and is getting acquainted with them, while the selling physician's role diminishes with a gradually curtailed workload.)

The agreement should specify the timeline of the sale. For example, some phase-out agreements last up to five years. If during that period the selling physician agrees to work three days a week and the buyer five days a week, this arrangement must be stated, with income allocations based on productivity and cost.

When executing the contract for the sale, purchasing physicians should place a designated percentage of the purchase price in escrow. Money should be added to the escrow fund annually. This fund will become the sellers' at the end of the phase-out period when the practice officially changes hands. The balance is then expended over time, typically a stipulated number of years. This procedure allows the selling physicians to defer income and thus gain some tax advantages. For retiring physicians whose income will drop sharply after retirement, the capital gains tax to be paid on the proceeds of the sale will be levied when the physicians are in a lower tax bracket.

Payment arrangements also are advantageous to purchasing physicians. Usually, purchasing physicians have limited resources available for purchasing the practice and likely have extended obligations, such as education loans repayment, a growing family, and mortgage payments, and cannot afford the expense of starting a solo practice.

The phase-out agreement should be well documented in a written contract. The contract should specify the following:

- All payment arrangements with exact specification of dollar amounts
- Time schedule including a firm phase-out date
- Allocations of total price to equipment, furnishings, patient records, supplies, goodwill, restrictive covenant, telephone number, leasehold improvements, and accounts receivable, if included in the sale
- Method of financing and percentage of ownership by each party
- Work hours, time off, vacation period, and other benefit-related agreements
- Personnel rules and regulations along with expected work load and work distribution
- A bill of sale for the tangible assets
- If applicable, the separation of real estate from other assets
- Elements pertinent to the sale, eg, parties to the agreement and the location of the practice
- A definite retirement date

A letter that announces the retirement is also useful (see Figure 1-6).

Conclusion

The landscape for selling physician practices has changed dramatically from that of even five to seven years ago. Nowadays, most practices are being sold to health systems or hospitals and entail very little, if any, upfront payment other than the fair market value of the tangible assets and perhaps the creation value of the medical records. Truly, the market for practices outside of health systems has diminished dramatically, likewise decreasing the strategies for selling physicians.

Most health systems and hospitals have an alignment strategy that involves a portion devoted to acquiring practices and employing physicians. This is specialty-specific, with some specialties in greater demand than others. Typically, the specialties that are in demand today are primary care, general surgery, cardiology, orthopedics, neurology, neurosurgery, and subspecialties of internal medicine and surgical subspecialties. Clinical areas such as dermatology, allergy, and others are not in great demand and would rarely be of interest to health systems unless their model is to employ all physicians within the community that are active within their medical staff. Some strategies like these exist.

As ACOs become more prevalent, and the model for subsequent payment structure for Medicare and, likely, private insurers, consolidation of medical practices with health systems or hospitals may become more predominant. Private practicing physicians will be in the minority, especially within urban and metropolitan areas where ACOs may be formed with greater flexibility.

Nonetheless, as physicians prepare to sell their practice, some matters have been applicable for many years, such as preparing the practice for sale and obtaining competent representation from both a health care consultant and health care specialized attorney, and are still necessary. Understanding the market and the structure of such transactions is also imperative. For example, knowing that currently very little (if any) goodwill is paid should not be a deterrent to a strategy that involves maximizing compensation to the physicians (within legal and regulatory parameters) over an extended period. The *value* of the practice realized in previous years as an upfront payment can be maximized over the life of the employment contract, especially when the new owner is a health system or hospital. While compensation structures are mostly tied to productivity requirements (as they should be), other upcoming payment forms include payment for quality and cost containment. These payments also will become a part of the compensation structure in the future. Compensation opportunities are available to offset the reduction in payment for the practice at the time of the transaction.

Smart owners should become smart sellers at some point. Being able to understand the market and the trends are imperative to being able to respond to both regulatory and market-driven terms and conditions.

Endnotes

1. Physician Services Payment System. Washington, DC: MEDPAC. Revised October 2010. http://www.medpac.gov/documents/MedPAC_Payment_Basics_10_Physician.pdf. Accessed May 25, 2011.
2. US Department of Health and Human Services, Centers for Medicare & Medicaid Services, Medicare Program; Medicare Shared Savings Program: Accountable Care Organizations, Proposed Rules. *Federal Register*, vol 76, No. 67, Thursday, April 7, 2011. http://edocket.access.gpo.gov/2011/pdf/2011-7880.pdf. Accessed May 25, 2011.
3. A New Approach to Patient Care: The Patient-Centered Medical Home. Washington, DC: Qualis Health. http://www.qhmedicalhome.org/. Accessed March 28, 2011.

CHAPTER 2 Disengagement

OUTLINE

In the current health care delivery environment, it is anticipated that some physicians who are employed by a hospital or contracted with a physician management company will likely fall victim to disengagement, the separation of employment. In fact, those that exceed an initial employment period beyond two or three years have probably worked through the nuances of a successful mutually beneficial relationship, meaning that they have learned to work together. For those who have not, disengagement has become a part of the physician practice in transition. (See Appendix A for additional resources that detail the disengagement process).

Characteristics of Disengagement

The decision to disengage is often jointly made by both the employer and the physician (employee). Obviously, the employer is either the hospital, management company, physician practice, or other entity that recruited and employed the physician or purchased the practice or subsequently "inherited" the physician as an employee. In a deteriorating relationship, for which disengagement is proposed, the employed physician is likely faced with going into private practice or finding another employed role. Either option represents a significant change both personally and professionally.

Hospitals and Health Systems

Many hospitals and health care systems are deciding whether to continue to support their employed physician networks or pursue some other alignment option. More and more systems are in the process of renegotiating physician contracts or at least restructuring compensation to be more productivity based and/or include patient satisfaction and quality indicators. They realize that the system as currently structured simply does not work, primarily because they purchased the practices for different reasons. For example, hospitals that purchased practices as a defensive measure may not have had the necessary resources and specific expertise to operate the practice. As a result, the compensation systems that were created, in effect, became disincentives to being productive.

In addition, hospitals have been dealing with numerous unfavorable payment structures (possibly even competing with the very physicians they wish to employ) due to restrictive managed care environments. This situation will most likely change with the use of a global payment or bundling process. As a result, hospitals are looking closer at the employment situation relative to physicians and structure. In cases in which physician goals are not aligned with corporate or system goals, the solution is disengagement.

Physician Practices

Most independent medical practices will continue to employ physicians, at least on an interim basis (until partnership eligibility is earned). However, the entire employment scenario is being carefully evaluated.

For example, some physician practices will employ physicians with the understanding that the arrangement is in effect more like a partnership, where involvement, compensation, and decision-making feedback are encouraged. In many situations, the partners are technically employees of the practice, but ultimately their compensation and their overall conduct, including administrative and management functions, are that of a partner.

Physician Practice Management Companies

The number of physician practice management companies (PPMCs), which once were common, has declined in recent years for various reasons, largely due to different goals and objectives. These changes have led to total restructuring or disengagement. Most recently, PPMCs have been replaced by management services organizations (MSO), co-management agreements, independent practice associations (IPA), revitalization, physician hospital organizations (PHO), and by early 2012, accountable care organizations (ACO). Those PPMCs that remain are reevaluating their entire structure and, for the most part, changing their business services and overall business plan to exclude the management of physicians.

Processes of Disengagement

The decision to disengage usually results when expectations and commitments made prior to affiliation are not fulfilled. Typically, these are manifested as decreased revenue or collections or reduced compensation. This section addresses the various options to consider in preparing for disengagement.

Deciding to Separate

The decision to separate from a hospital, physician practice, or management company can be a life-changing decision that affects physicians (and their families) personally as well as professionally. The decision typically results when promises and commitments made prior to entering into the affiliation are not fulfilled. It may also arise when physicians notice the impact of declining payments in a market at the same time as their respective overhead expenditures continue to increase.

The decision to disengage involves many options and questions. The following questions should be considered in this process:

- Are the physicians' and organization's mission, values, and vision congruent?

- What are the financial implications of discontinuing the affiliation?
- What are the immediate and long-term financial implications of remaining in the current affiliation?
- What impact would reductions in payment have on the relationship?
- Have the network's or group's accounts payable increased dramatically in recent months as a result of tighter cash flows?
- Has the corporation withheld salary or bonus payments to the partners or providers (again, possibly due to cash flow challenges)?
- How will the competition respond to the disengagement?
- How will the community respond to the disengagement?
- How will other physicians and referral relationships be affected by the decision to terminate the relationship?
- What will be the impact on patient satisfaction?
- How will payers respond?
- What will have to be done to minimize short-term negative publicity and help communicate the overall benefits of the process?
- Is there a restrictive covenant in the physician contract, and will it have an impact on the physician's ability to practice?
- If the practice is to exist post-disengagement, what operational and financial changes will have to be made?

From the physician's perspective, re-entering private practice in the community or entering private practice for the first time brings numerous challenges and opportunities, all of which require significant time and resources. Many of the challenges are similar to those experienced when starting a practice. The following is a list of these challenges:

- Developing a customized pro forma/business plan to attain financing to purchase the practice as well as for ongoing day-to-day operational expenditures
- Developing a competitive fee schedule and payment strategy
- Negotiating or renegotiating managed care and vendor contracts
- Identifying and selecting health care benefits and other benefits for the practice
- Establishing proper protocols for medical records, including the current electronic health record (EHR) initiatives
- Assessing appropriate space requirements and relocation of office space in the community
- Developing and filing corporate documents for the new legal entity

- Obtaining new provider numbers
- Restoring a practice billing office operation or central billing office (CBO) participation
- Developing an appropriate management team on either an interim or a permanent basis
- Selecting an appropriate information and financial system with installation and training
- Developing and implementing a practice compliance plan
- Training and organizing staff
- Developing practice policies and procedures manuals

In addition, a physician may choose to become employed by another entity rather than open a private practice. A few questions to consider here include:

- What are the expectations of the new employer and how do they differ from the prior one?
- What are the physician's expectations as to quality of life, work schedule, call coverage, and compensation?
- How significant is the benefits structure?
- Will the management structure support an environment that allows the physician to attain both productivity and non-productivity goals?
- How strong is the physician leadership team and do the members have similar quality and practice styles?

Phases of Disengagement under a Repurchase Arrangement

Disengagements from hospital networks and from physician practices are distinctly different due to their inherent nature and the relationship among the parties after separation. As the components of the separation process are defined, depending on the circumstances, it is important to assign tasks among internal staff, external and internal consultants, and attorneys. The key to success is to have a workable plan with specific responsibilities and guidelines as well as developed timelines. This approach will lead to a clear plan that involves all applicable parties. The following sections detail the key phases of disengagement.

Phase 1: Conceptual Modeling

The first step in the disengagement process is to accumulate organizational, operational, and financial data to be used in the unwinding process. By definition, the unwinding process encompasses the functions of separating the physician previously employed or subject to a management agreement from the employer or management company. Typically, this includes a due diligence review that is performed by an independent consultant. When appropriate, attorneys should work closely with the consultant. Thus the team for the unwinding process is made up of these outside experts and the physicians, with participation from representatives of the employer or management company.

The feasibility of unwinding should be considered at this phase. Certain practices in a hospital network will want divestiture and others will want to continue in the employment arrangement. The hospital must keep in mind the importance of maintaining its relationship with the physicians, whether they are employed or move to a private practice. This consideration includes other referral sources and proper specialty coverage.

Conceptual modeling at this phase calls for both on- and off-site work, preferably by an independent third party. Phase one includes meeting with the physicians to apprise them of the unwinding process and establishing a solid foundation for both parties. It also entails an on-site operational assessment plus an independent valuation of the practice. The independent third party will prepare a formal written report and offer recommendations. The conclusions will be based on these reviews relative to the due diligence of the practice and the independent valuation.

After completing phase one, the team working on the unwinding process will interview key physicians and management and start disseminating information from the report. Presentations to the physicians will be completed, and the physicians will be presented with a definite plan of action for the unwinding process.

Phase 2: Negotiating Repurchase and Starting the Transition

Phase two entails time to review, digest, and agree on the independent valuation and operational assessment of the practice review that was done during phase one. Legal analysis will also be completed. If the entire practice must be repurchased, fair market value (FMV) and negotiations cannot favor either party, especially when a hospital is involved in the transaction.

Unwinding a management company is a somewhat different process because it may be based on a negotiated settlement. If the physicians wish to leave the management company, the basis for the negotiations is the independent consultant's analysis and due diligence review of the operations and the negotiated value of the assets being repurchased.

Phase two also includes final negotiations and reaching an agreed upon price. When a hospital unwinds a practice and sells it back to the physicians, the sale will most likely be subject to FMV regulations. Issues about current value, which may be much less than the original selling price, should be resolved, and an agreement for reacquisition obtained. A significant element of the FMV process is that of assessing and independently valuing tangible assets. In a number of situations, the resulting value can be unfavorably affected due to fully depreciated assets that carry no (or limited) value. Competent health care attorneys should be involved in this stage of the disengagement process to draft the proper legal agreements and assist in executing the documents. After that process is complete, the transition process begins.

Phase 3: Reorganization Implementation

The transition process for an entire practice is followed by actual implementation of the new practice's operations. Certain tasks (provided in the following list) must be completed during the transition prior to actual repurchase or privatization. Other tasks, such as transfer of medical records, lease and other contract assignments, official termination, and rehiring of employees, should not be separated and should not be done until the repurchase transaction is complete. Normally, this transaction is memorialized for the entire practice through an asset purchase agreement (APA), which outlines the terms and conditions and the items that are purchased within the transaction.

The reorganization phase may last from three to five months, and will entail some or all of the following activities:

- Formation of the new legal entities, possibly including newly acquired provider numbers
- Reestablishment of centralized services, ie, management and administration
- Appointment of an interim management team or outsourcing of management to an independent practice management entity
- Establishing support systems, eg, information systems and financial systems
- Hiring and training staff
- Defining policies and procedures
- Reviewing and entering vendor contracts
- Reviewing and entering important managed care organization (MCO) agreements
- Designing employee benefit programs

Phase 4: Post-Unwind Support

The final phase, post-unwind support, may not be necessary in certain instances. For example, practices that separate from a management company will obtain little, if any, support in the unwinding process. Hospital networks may provide some assistance, especially for day-to-day management, and continue to lease property and needed assistance. Obviously, everything must be at a fair market price and in a legal and compliant manner.

Specific areas in which post-unwind support may be necessary include:

- Managerial system audits
- Compliance support
- Human resources
- Physician recruitment
- Operations, marketing, and managed care support
- Merger and acquisition opportunity evaluation

Legal Issues

Key legal issues prevail in the process of disengaging physicians, including disengagements from hospitals, physician practices, and management companies. Management agreements from management companies usually contain a section on the obligations of both parties on termination of the agreement. In general, the agreement provides that the physician group must repurchase the assets used in the operations of the physician group, and it will be specific as to the methodology for determining the purchase price of those assets.

After the assets are repurchased by the physician group, the management agreement should be terminated. The physician group is then free to conduct its medical practice separate and apart from the management company. Specific issues to consider in the termination process are as follows:

- Accounts receivable
- Bank relationships
- Personnel
- Assumption of contracts
- Repurchase of assets
- Purchase price for assets

In addition, all these matters must be considered in the transitional process to assure an effective privatization.

Unlike management companies, hospitals must strictly adhere to legal requirements of the disengagement process. Three primary legal issues that affect nearly every aspect of the divestiture process are the anti-kickback statute, the Stark Law, and, for tax-exempt institutions, the prohibition of inurement, the prohibition against excessive private benefit, and intermediate sanction rules.

The anti-kickback statute prohibits, among other things, the payment of anything of value to a referral source in return for the referral from or to a business reimbursable by a governmental program such as Medicare. The statute's scope is comprehensive, and the courts have not hesitated to apply it broadly.

The Stark Law prohibits a physician from making a referral to a provider for the furnishing of "designated health services" reimbursable by Medicare or Medicaid if the physician has a financial relationship with the provider, unless an exception applies. The term *designated health services* is specifically confined to this regulation; overall, it includes virtually any inpatient and outpatient hospital services. Accordingly, unless an exception exists, physicians are unable to make any referrals to their former employer after the transition.

There are two methods for ensuring access to an exception. First, the unwind can be viewed as simply a modification of a set of existing agreements, each of which may have its own exception. Second, there is an exception under the Stark statute for *isolated transactions*. In general, a transaction is an isolated transaction if the amounts to be paid to the physician are consistent with FMV, they are not determined in a manner that takes into account the volume or value of any referrals, and the payments are made pursuant to an agreement that would be commercially reasonable even if no referrals were made. *Private inurement, private benefit,* and *intermediate sanctions rules* apply to tax-exempt entities or entities that include a tax-exempt entity within an integrated delivery system.

1. First, the tax-exempt employer must take care to avoid violating the prohibition against private inurement. Health care facilities that have been recognized by the Internal Revenue Service (IRS) as a tax-exempt entity must be concerned about remaining tax-exempt under their appropriate taxation code. They may do this if no part of their net earnings inures to the benefit of a private shareholder or an individual who has a personal and private interest in the activities of a tax-exempt organization, sometimes referred to as *insiders*.

2. Second, the IRS has developed another guideline for determining the worthiness of a tax-exempt entity. This guideline is generally referred to as the private benefit test. The tax-exempt status may be lost if the private benefit conferred on the individual outweighs the public benefit enjoyed by the institution and the community.

3. Finally, when divesting themselves of private practices, a tax-exempt organization must consider that, until recently, the only enforcement tool available to the IRS in connection with such a violation was a revocation of the tax exemption. Now, intermediate sanctions can be authorized. The IRS can impose an excise tax on certain individuals, referred to as disqualified persons,

involved in a transaction in which the individual receives an economic benefit from an exempt organization that exceeds the value of consideration provided to such organizations, such as the sale of a physician practice. This could be construed as acceptable, if the terms of the sale result in the organization receiving less than FMV.

Specific components of the divestiture process include termination of the employment agreement and transfer of assets to the physicians. Both have several component parts that should be considered and dealt with in the divestiture process.

Valuation and Negotiations

The independent valuation of the practice must be done for legal purposes, especially if it involves a hospital. The valuation should be completed as a part of the due diligence process and, accordingly, should include an operational assessment of the practice. This assessment will enable the prospective new owner or physician to understand its operations. It also forms the basis for the calculations and conclusions of the valuation, resulting in a formal report. The valuation should be prepared by a qualified independent party knowledgeable in practice operations and the valuation processes. This valuator should understand the approaches to valuation and apply these as applicable. (See Appendix A for resources that discuss the proper approach to performing a valuation.)

It is best to establish the value of the practice based on its reacquisition by the original physician owner who was employed by the hospital, independent practice, or management company after its sale. The owners of the asset prior to its original sale or acquisition recognize the true value of these assets. However, the value of the practice could be significantly different upon reacquisition. For most hospitals that are divesting themselves of ownership, the value of the practice at divestiture is significantly less than what it was worth during the original purchase. This reduction is generally due to a decrease in productivity and a potential increase in expenses. In fact, the very reason for the divestiture may be less than acceptable operating results. This scenario is typical now, as usually only tangible assets are involved.

The reason for an independent appraisal is to help establish a fair and balanced value. As mentioned, the FMV appraisal is necessary due to legal and governmental guidelines. Thus, the parties ideally should agree ahead of time to have the independent appraisal and accept the appraiser's conclusion of value to reduce the amount of negotiations.

Absent an agreement to concur on an independent appraisal, the parties must agree to the negotiation, terms, and conditions of the sale, which relies on the overall willingness of the parties to complete the disengagement process.

Part of the valuation process involves negotiating the purchase price. In brief, if a hospital is selling the practice, the total FMV, as assigned by the independent appraiser, would subsequently become the agreed upon price. There should be very little change to this total unless certain assets are eliminated or other matters relative to the valuator's assumptions are legitimately adjusted. In such cases, the valuator will need to update or change the conclusions and adjust the valuation totals.

Private physicians who are considering a repurchase of their practice from a private group or management company have more flexibility regarding purchase price negotiations. Although the independent appraisal should be the benchmark on which the negotiations rest, the actual transaction value can be less, or perhaps even more, than the valuation total. It would be rare for the transaction value to be greater than the independent valuation total, but it is possible if the parties legitimately include additional components that enhance the value.

Specific assets that will be purchased (or not purchased) as well as liabilities that may be assumed are part of the negotiation as well. For example, the former owner may choose to maintain ownership of the accounts receivable, or they could be sold to the new physician owner.

Most practices do not want tangible assets separated when the practice is sold. Prospective buyers are expected to take on all assets. The independent valuator should consider the assets as one unit and function, as such, with the valuation including the assets as a total package and not valued individually. This method commonly results in a higher value than if the assets had been individually valued. Other assets that may be part of the transaction should be specifically identified and negotiated.

Liabilities may be assumed, depending on the structure of the transition. Obviously, any liabilities assumed would offset or reduce the actual net purchase amount that is paid at closing. Contingent liabilities should be identified and negotiated, with a clear understanding that if they result, the selling practice would be responsible for making the buyer financially whole. Such contingent liabilities, if realized, should be accounted for between the buyer and the seller, with the seller giving credit (or direct payment) to the buyer for them.

Goodwill and other intangible assets, for example, trademarks, patents, royalty arrangements, and other areas of potential intangible worth, may be identified by the independent valuator. These intangible assets are subject to negotiations between the buyer and seller and can be included in the transaction or negotiated out, in certain instances. Often, the name of the selling practice will have accrued value in the community, becoming a trade name of sorts. While the name may have some value, the purchasing physician does not necessarily have to buy it, assuming that the new practice will operate under a different name.

The recent trend has been to avoid the valuation of intangible assets because of the difficulty in deriving an agreed upon calculation. Typical with any sales transaction, a seller commonly believes the value of its entity to be higher, while a buyer is unwilling to see an increased value due to uncertainties and unknown risks.

Privatization Process

Within the privatization process, there are three major areas to consider: (1) reestablishment of the practice to its prior state or as a newly formed private entity, (2) the implementation of a plan to complete this, and (3) the actual transitioning processes.

Reestablishing the Practice

Reestablishment of the practice is indeed a major challenge, no matter what the prior setting. Hospitals that are in a disengagement process from physicians have limitations as to what is legally appropriate in assisting with the reestablishment of a practice. A health system can help sell the practice at a fair market value and assist in specific operational transitioning, but it must first obtain a legal opinion from a health care attorney.

Often, an independent consultant can play a key role in guiding the parties through the transition to avoid legal pitfalls. The physicians may be obligated to pay for certain services, but the health system can assist within the legal framework of the disengagement process. The physicians of the health system should explore how and to what extent the health system can assist within these legal parameters.

A PPMC disengagement is not subject to the same legal scrutiny, so there is more flexibility. However, the PPMC will likely be unwilling to assist in the reestablishment for simple economic and relational reasons.

In the final analysis, the new physician owners are responsible for establishing their practice. Figure 2-1 lists the key responsibilities that they need to consider.

A good way to start reorganization and reestablishment is through a committee structure. If the new practice is large and the transition involves several physicians from a hospital network or PPMC to a single or multispecialty private group, sub-departmental organization may be appropriate. Specific roles may be assigned to the following categories:

- Securing operating capital, financing asset repurchase
- Assessing information technology, including financial and practice management systems and electronic health records
- Implementing a governance structure for the reorganized group
- Recruiting a practice management team, either for an interim or a full-time basis
- Developing a strategic plan for long term and a business plan for the near term
- Drafting retirement and benefit goals and objectives
- Developing a compliance plan

FIGURE 2-1 Key Responsibilities

- Information technology
- Financial and revenue cycle management
- Human resources and personnel matters
- Governance, leadership, and management structure
- Marketing and managed care contracting strategy
- Operations, including policies and procedures and day-to-day administrative management
- Quality assurance, including establishing clinical standards and protocols

Implementing the Plan

The actual implementation process may span several months. Although support may not be provided by the health system or the PPMC, certain individuals from outside the system may help the practice initially plan the implementation and identify a qualified outside consultant who can facilitate and assist in many areas. If the PPMC disengagement is reasonably amenable, the PPMC may assist in linking the new entity with a qualified consultant and even coordinating some of the functions.

Reorganization and implementation of the practice consists of many of the actions outlined previously in the chapter.

If the physician or practice conducts it own implementation process, the transition is performed by a combination of individuals: the new physician owners, the new internal management, and, as appropriate, external consultants and attorneys. This team approach to the transition, if given a sufficient amount of time, should result in a well-established newly privatized entity.

The matter of time is significant. Normally, at least 6 months, and preferably 9 to 12 months, from the very beginning of the disengagement process is needed to complete the transitioning process. While it could be done faster, it would have to be a highly organized, well-managed process to be carried out in such a short period. Realistically, this accelerated timeline is not normally achieved, especially if frustrations and, to some extent, tenuous relations have developed between the physician owners and their employer or contractor (ie, the health system, PPMC, or private group).

Managing the Transition

The transitioning period is essential to the success of the newly privatized practice. Physicians who have been out of private practice for years may be returning reluctantly. Others may never have been in private practice, so this whole experience is new. Whatever their previous background, physicians must understand how to operate a private business. In effect, the major purposes of the transitioning practice are to help physicians understand what it is like to practice as a private enterprise and to complete the necessary processes to assure success in this new business endeavor.

In general, the difference between a successful transition and an unsuccessful one involves the handling of personnel and other human resource issues. Employees of the group in transition are understandably concerned with matters as immediate as their next paycheck to longer term issues such as retirement benefits, health insurance, and general job stability. It is thus important to focus on retaining employees through the transition by ensuring that personnel issues are handled appropriately.

Managing through the transition process to independence requires constant attention to all details of practice operations from the clinical to the administrative. A poorly planned and executed transition can have enormous financial ramifications. Its impact on the future of the practice is likewise immense. Thus, the stage is set from the beginning for success or failure.

To address the transition plan, use a disengagement and transition plan checklist as provided in *Beyond Disengagement: Recreating the Physician Practice.*[1] This checklist lists the issues related to the areas of responsibility for both hospitals and PPMCs in the unwinding process. Physicians should develop their own checklist and work with individuals who have an understanding of each component. The transition process should therefore include the items outlined in Figure 2-2. Within these items, a timeline should be established for the completion of each area of responsibility. Likewise, individuals should be assigned roles to each of those areas.

The transition plan may be completed in a relatively short time under certain circumstances. A PPMC transition process is usually accomplished fairly quickly, in that the PPMC does relatively little to support the newly privatized practice after the actual assets are purchased and the liabilities are assumed. Once the decision is made, the PPMC sells the assets as negotiated back to the physicians. The physicians are then left with the immediate responsibilities of management and operations. This process results in a brief window of time, sometimes no more than 60 to 90 days.

With a hospital or health system disengagement, the health system should employ a qualified health care consultant to assist the physician (primarily converting operational functions from network to private practice). Realistically, this process could take a reasonable amount of time, perhaps as long as 6 to 12 months.

In summary, a smooth transition involves many initiatives (see Figure 2-3), yet it should be completed by the date that was originally set. As timelines and responsibilities are outlined and assigned, the process can be completed with efficiency and effectiveness.

- Reviewing the historical operating data to prepare for the independent valuation and/or due diligence process to derive a repurchase amount
- Reviewing different physician issues (including assignment or confirmation of a lease agreement, termination of employment terms, practice insurance assignment or new policy, and determination of retirement termination funds and the correlated disposition of them)
- Defining personnel functions
- Making the transition from employee benefit programs
- Managing licensing arrangements
- Attending to other matters, whether they relate to day-to-day operations or more closely involve the physicians' practice functions that are part of the transitioning process

FIGURE 2-2 Disengagement/Transition Plan Checklist

- Developing information technology and financial systems
- Coordinating purchasing
- Developing a staffing model
- Transitioning the retirement benefit plan
- Restoring and reestablishing a central billing office
- Developing and implementing a compliance plan
- Transferring managed care and vendor contracts
- Performing all other operations

FIGURE 2-3 Smooth Transition

Residual Relationships

Ideally, the disengaging partners are forming residual or new relationships after the employment relationship is terminated. It is hoped that the physicians will remain members of the hospital's medical staff, function on various medical staff committees, and work diligently within that hospital facility through their inpatient practice, and perhaps some outpatient services (performed within the hospital). Thus, clearly there is a need for both parties to maintain a civil relationship, even if employment has changed.

Although someone might initially think that very little, if any, residual relationships could result after a PPMC disengagement, this is seldom the case. Some PPMCs will continue to provide management services to the practice after the disengagement has occurred. Still others are developing new service lines that actually call for a continued working relationship with the practice. For example, a major PPMC, US Oncology Network, is developing a pharmaceutical service line, using a process whereby they will contract with formerly managed practices for the purchase of pharmaceuticals (eg, for drug infusion therapy) to that oncology practice.

Thus, no matter what the feelings and the reasons are for the disengagement, it is important that the two parties try to work through their differences during the reestablishment and transition stages, particularly if they envision working together afterward.

It is also important to maintain good relationships within the community and with the patients that are served. Neither party benefits if patients believe that there is hostility between the physicians and the hospital, particularly as a former employer. It is best for both parties to get along throughout the entire disengagement process.

Often, the physicians and the former employer work much better together after the employment relationship is terminated. Although they may operate at arm's length, they still can work collaboratively in such a way that goals and positive operating results are achieved. Overall, the community usually benefits the most from this cooperation, as it is advantageous for physicians and hospitals to work together to better serve the community.

Conclusion

Physicians who are employed by a hospital or who have contracted with a physician management company will likely undergo the process of disengagement as a part of the ongoing transitions in health care. The better prepared all the parties involved are in this process, the better the outcomes and ongoing relationships will be in the delivery of health care.

Endnote

1. Reiboldt JM, Hunter CW. *Beyond Disengagement—Recreating the Physician Practice.* Chicago: American Medical Association; 2001:44–9.

CHAPTER 3 Physician Diversification

OUTLINE

I. Introduction
II. Alternatives to the Traditional Business Model
   A. Adding Ancillary Services
   B. Adding Partners
   C. Additional Ventures
III. Business Opportunities
   A. Thinking Retail
   B. New Revenue Opportunities
   C. Retail Strategies
IV. The Possibilities of Partnering
   A. Partnership Evaluation Facets: Relational
   B. Partnership Evaluation Facets: Financial
   C. Failed Partnerships
   D. Alternative Collaborations
V. The Political Fallout
VI. Legal Constraints and Considerations
VII. Conclusion

As reductions in payment continue to place more and more pressure on the medical practice, the basic business model of the traditional medical practice is changing. Many physicians are realizing that to enhance their personal wealth through their business, they must consider alternative models to the traditional outpatient medical practice. Depending on the specialty, there are opportunities to build value and increase overall profitability by diversifying.

Many physicians believe that diversification requires some sort of professional affiliation. Others find the intrusion of business issues and risk into the practice as offensive. Yet, many physicians today are aggressively seeking opportunities to build lucrative business ventures within the context of their given medical specialty and training. To assure a good fit within the organization's business model and with its physicians, professional values and personal temperament are key to successful diversification. As part of the review of the medical practice in transition, it is important to evaluate the alternatives and the possibilities pertaining to such diversification.

Alternatives to the Traditional Business Model

By definition, a business model encompasses the size, structure, and services of a practice or other health care entity. This business model can be changed in many ways. For example, some practices increase their size by adding physicians or merging with other practices. Others achieve business diversification by forming separate entities so that they can invest in ancillary services and facilities. For example, a group of surgeons who own their own individually managed outpatient practices may come together to form a new company that invests in and owns ancillary ventures such as an ambulatory service center (ASC). Other physicians from specialties such as orthopedics, otolaryngology, urology, ophthalmology, general surgery, pain management, gynecology, and gastroenterology may build and operate an ASC (see Figure 3-1). This arrangement opens up a new area of financial opportunity, because the ASC does not generate revenue from professional charges. Rather it generates income from the technical and facility fees.

Adding Ancillary Services

Although incorporating ancillary services or an ancillary venture into the overall business model may require a separate legal entity, it can be a viable business venture that complements, even augments, the basic practice. Such diversification comes with a great deal of risk, including managed care and payment, demographic makeup, financial strength of the local economy, and imbalances between supply and demand for comparable services. These risks must be evaluated and measured by the diversified physician-owned organization and addressed within its overall business strategy. Physicians must be willing to accept the worst outcomes from these risks, including loss of income.

Of course, diversification does come with rewards, including increased personal income and net worth and improved quality of life. Often, surgeons express frustration with the lack of control they have over scheduling the operating room facilities at the local hospital. After constructing their own ASC, they have much more flexibility. This flexibility leads to greater efficiency not only within the ASC but also within their own outpatient practice.

Specialty	Ancillary Venture
Anesthesiology/pain management	Ambulatory service center (ASC)
Cardiology	Catheterization laboratory
Dermatology	Surgery center
Endocrinology	Nutrition center/health education
Family practice	Laboratory and diagnostic wellness centers
Gastroenterology	ASC/endoscopy center
Hematology/oncology	Cancer center including radiation oncology
Infectious disease	Laboratory diagnostic wellness centers
Internal medicine	Laboratory diagnostic subspecialty ventures
Nephrology	Renal center
Obstetrician/gynecologist	Surgery center
Ophthalmology	Surgery center, optical shop
Pediatrics	Diagnostic and laboratory center
Podiatry	Surgery center
Pulmonary medicine	Sleep centers
General surgery	Surgery center
Plastic and reconstructive surgery	Surgery center
Urgent care	Walk-in clinic, urgent care center
Urology	Continence center, surgery center
Orthopedic surgery	Surgery center
Plastic and reconstructive surgery	Surgery center

FIGURE 3-1 Commonplace Ancillary Ventures by Specialty

Another reward comes from the physicians' ability to expand their presence throughout the community for the delivery of health care services. Physicians who traditionally looked to the local hospital for support in these ventures can gain independence, reap the benefits of such diversification, and still stay within their level of clinical expertise.

Adding Partners

Alternatively, many physicians diversify by adding partners. This arrangement mitigates the risk and allows for a more communal attitude toward the delivery of care. In many instances, the physician partners with a local hospital(s). For the community's long-term welfare, it is best that both physicians and hospitals be successful.

Problems can occur for any business when it strays too far from its core competency or adds too many services that cause it to fragment and lose focus. These same problems can occur for physicians or hospitals that try to provide too many services without the proper backup, expertise, infrastructure, and staffing. In some cases, a partnership between a physician and hospital may be a solution worth exploring before investing in a new service. However, it can be a challenge to join hospitals and independent physicians in such a venture. With the advent of accountable care organizations (ACO), this kind of diversification will likely occur more frequently.

Additional Ventures

Moreover, real estate opportunities, such as medical office buildings and other facilities that are technically outside of the realm of the day-to-day physician practice, offer additional areas of diversification. These areas truly qualify as diversification, even though they are somewhat outside of the immediate realm of clinical expertise (transcending to real estate management).

The many alternatives to the traditional business model available to the physician must be evaluated and weighed in the balance as they relate to the following:

- Overall impact on the community
- Relational impact between the—
  - physician and other physicians
  - physician and the hospitals
  - physician and the community at large
- Financial return on investment
- Legal requirements relative to physicians investing in such health care entities

Business Opportunities

One of the biggest challenges for any physician is to expand a business. What strategies are available for physicians to do this? If physicians are devoted only to their outpatient practice, the limitations for growth are apparent. Physicians can either work longer hours or expand to new locations, additional providers, and the like. Obviously, these options come with added cost and increased risk. There also is the question of viability, because the market for such traditional services is mature and spending is, in fact, decreasing. In addition, physicians must decide about making a reinvestment in the practice infrastructure, including information technology. Physicians must constantly weigh the costs of meeting social and community service goals against the reward of being involved in such activities. Time taken to branch out and expand a business must come from somewhere, and the needs of the community or a physicians' social network should be assessed.

Expanding a business is a challenge, because most approaches to grow revenue lack creativity and fail to take advantage of emerging technology and consumer trends and demands. Most physicians focus instead on capturing shrinking premium dollars and market shares for their individual practice. This approach perpetuates a "sickness" model, even while the population around them is more concerned about wellness and maintaining health. To avoid such stagnation, many physicians are thinking retail.

Thinking Retail

Webster's defines retail as "the sale of commodities or goods in small quantities to ultimate consumers."[1] Thinking retail involves taking the perspective of the consumer, in this case patients, and developing service features and attributes that will prompt the consumer to purchase directly from the business owner, the physicians. Of course, many traditional health services will continue (perhaps always) to be sold through wholesaling intermediaries (ie, insurance and managed care companies). However, physicians should not assume that it is no longer important to seek good managed care contracts with insurance companies. Rather, that is just one of many components in the process of customer acquisition and retention.

The historical orientation of facility-based providers and the traditional system of payment focus on large-scale purchasers. These entities include the federal government (Medicare), state and local governments (Medicaid), private third parties mostly through insurance companies, and managed care organizations. The insurers have consolidated, and the government entities continue to provide payment in ever-diminishing returns. Thus, more and more pressure exists for providers of health care, in this case, physicians.

Unfortunately, physicians usually say that they have little control over the services they provide; it is the health plans, including government payers, that dictate what will be reimbursed. In many marketplaces, this approach has led to the view of traditional health care services as a commodity. As a result, many ancillary ventures that focus in certain specific areas have been developed, similar to those discussed earlier that relate to ancillary ventures of individual physicians. Private for-profit companies have also approached physicians in an aggressive manner. The concept of thinking "retail" about the business has thus evolved. Without intending to minimize the importance and the overall priority of physicians to provide quality health care (and to care about their patients), this business approach must be considered.

Many medical care organizations, such as health maintenance organizations (HMO) and preferred provider organizations (PPO), are unable to provide the consumer with quality service, such as the ability to obtain appointments or provide short waiting times. Of course, cost or price is also a factor.

A number of socioeconomic trends are promoting this move to a more retail-oriented marketplace, including changing populations, technology, and the cost of health care. Opportunities exist to sell preventive screening services (diabetes, cancer), improve home accessibility and functionality, conduct support groups, sell information on social and medical services, provide cosmetic pharmaceuticals and vitamins, and even provide housing and living alternatives, all within the framework of delivering health care. The largest demographic group, the "baby boomers" (born between 1945 and 1964), is now also the biggest block of the population, which influences the consumption of health care, especially as this population ages. Baby boomers have traditionally valued convenience, control, and customer service. They do not hesitate to obtain alternative services or find different ways to obtain health care, particularly if it means better service for the cost.

New Revenue Opportunities

Physicians interested in entering the retail market could likely sell expanded services to the growing baby-boomer population, such as the following: self-help books and tapes; computer-oriented educational programs; quick tests for blood pressure level and other health status indicators at shopping malls; and alternative therapies such as massage, biofeedback, and acupuncture. In addition, so-called boutique medicine is appearing in certain markets. These arrangements entail a select number of patients paying physicians an annual fee for full and complete access to services (relatively on demand). Other physicians are taking their practice to the patient. For example, physicians may go to a business person's office or home to treat basic cold or flu symptoms.

The penchant many aging baby boomers have for a youthful appearance has stimulated demand for many physician services. Cosmetic surgeries, such as tummy tucks, vein treatment, hair replacement, facelifts, and other cosmetic procedures, are being performed in non-clinical settings and essentially are paid out-of-pocket on a fee-for-service basis.

The tremendous technological advances that have been introduced in the marketplace in the past few decades offer new revenue opportunities. They provide enhancements through information access, self-diagnosis, and even home-testing facilities. The ability to measure cholesterol, blood glucose, and protein levels; test for human immunodeficiency virus (HIV) and pregnancy; and even help parents diagnose ear infections have grown into a major industry.

Currently, researchers are working on ways to detect other diseases such as strep throat, ulcers, and even venereal disease. Interactive systems take blood pressure and pulse and monitor medication usage, making self-care or home health care feasible for the chronically ill and attractive for their caregivers.

The emerging media and marketplace of the Internet is certain to offer opportunities in retail markets from remote diagnosis to help via chat rooms for persons with chronic or acute illnesses.

While not all of these ventures have applicability to physicians, many do. Moreover, physicians must be savvy, understanding that they are a part of the overall health care delivery system. Physicians must have a heightened awareness of innovations and be willing to receive them into their practice as a viable alternative to more traditional procedures. Ultimately, these advances may provide better and more efficient services to patients at an effectively lower cost.

Retail Strategies

Retailing methodologies also apply to the way health care is presented to the marketplace. For example, some health care providers have minimized the importance of facility aesthetics, environment, and surroundings when treating patients. Believing that the health care environment is unimportant severely limits opportunity and growth. Today, many physicians are thinking more about facility convenience, accessibility, and aesthetics to make the overall practice experience more pleasant (realizing the limitations relative to a patient's degree of illness). Such improvements do not have to cost a lot; high-quality customer service often imparts the best "environment" of all. Simple, efficient personal registration processes; waiting rooms that appear more like a fine hotel's private sitting area than a seating area at an airport gate; access to comfort facilities such as restrooms and refreshments; accessibility to easy-to-understand information about the procedures, processes, and schedules of the patient encounter; and additional patient instructions and aids are all simple ways to improve the overall patient experience.

Another retail strategy is to offer related products and services to stimulate additional spending. Although this may be perceived as taboo, it is very much a part of today's medical experience. For example, expectant mothers will soon need to select a pediatrician or a family practitioner for newborn care. What process does the obstetrician use to help her make that selection? Primary care physicians often advise their patients on dieting and wellness. Another way to follow through on this role is to provide nutritional counseling services in the office,

Diversification is a fact of life in today's marketplace. For example, two successful retailers, Wal-Mart and Home Depot, are extremely diversified. The way to apply this success to health care is to look at business opportunities from the patient's point of view. For example, what types of health care services are available for adolescents who believe they are too old to see a pediatrician but cannot relate to their parent's general practitioners? There is obviously a niche to be addressed in this and many other areas of the medical practice.

The Possibilities of Partnering

Many reasons exist for aligning with other providers, including the following:

- Strength in numbers
- Creating a name-brand identity
- Assuring a cost-effective provider
- Diversification of payers (spread out the payer mix)
- Expansion of patient bases

This list represents basic yet very real reasons for forming such strategically aligned organizations.

There are several possibilities for partnering among physicians and ancillary or diversified ventures. The most logical is for fellow providers or physicians to come together in such a venture. Occasionally, physicians find partners in non-physician entities or individuals; these partnerships often take the form of joint ventures between physicians and hospitals.

Partnership Evaluation Facets: Relational

Each partnership should be evaluated to make sure it is a good fit for all involved. This fit is not always based on the financial or fiscal ramifications of the partnership. Considerations to be evaluated include the following:

- Attributes of potential partners
- Community orientation
- Ability to develop links with other health care providers
- Ability to develop an integrated information system
- Effectiveness in negotiating managed care contracts
- Capital investment potential
- Profitability potential
- Expense reduction potential

- Cultural compatibility
- Ability to achieve the goals of the partnership

Partnership Evaluation Facets: Financial

Areas that should be assessed to ensure that the partnership makes good business sense include the following:

- Fundamentally solid fiscal base
- Realistic strategic plan with a sound feasibility study
- Ability to expand
- Adequate community involvement
- Strong market penetration
- Cultural fit and willingness of physicians to work together
- Strategically viable location (both physically and within the practice structure) in the community

Moreover, any proposed joint venture or partnership should include the following:

- Purpose of the partnership
- Legal structure
- Assets/liabilities
- Governance
- Management
- Valuation
- Profit and loss sharing
- Capitalization/working capital
- Human resources
- Partnership exit
- Covenants to not compete
- Tax-exemption issues if applicable

Failed Partnerships

Despite efforts to create the ideal partnership, some mergers or partnerships fail. Usually, they fail when there is a lack of planning and coordination, eg, making key strategic decisions after the partnership has been formed. Other times partnerships fail because they are thought to be the ultimate solution but end up not solving all the existing problems. There may be clashes at the highest levels of the organization, or physicians are not able to get along and work together. Control is also a major factor. Some physicians give up control when they take on an equity partner and are simply not ready to do this.

When is the best time to create a partnership or joint venture? Usually, when two partners who are both financially stable are able to take the time to look for the right opportunity and to put together a well-planned and coordinated initiative. The ability to assess organizational strengths and weaknesses and acquire partners who will be strong contributors to the organization are also important for success. Of course, physicians who are willing to work together and truly function as partners will assure the success of the organization.

Alternative Hospital Collaborations

Although many physicians would prefer to be independent, partnerships and joint ventures are not always the best options. It may be somewhat difficult to accept, but the better alignment model for a physician may be with a hospital. However, hospitals and physicians participating in integrated delivery systems should realize that success cannot be achieved independent of each other. While the dynamics of physician employment by hospitals is changing, physicians and hospitals are working collaboratively to benefit both parties in the marketplace. As outlined in Chapter 1, such an arrangement may offer advantages.

In addition, there are strategic reasons for maintaining collaborative initiatives. Increased understanding of the market through broad-based services gives increased visibility in the community to both the physician and the hospital. More comprehensive services may also be the result. Another viable reason for joining forces is to pursue opportunities through consolidated systems to negotiate contracts. Last, another reason to partner is to attract quality managers and physicians in a desired practice setting for new physicians.

The overriding principles of physician integration should include a shared mission and values, structure that will thrive in a managed care environment (especially in capitation arrangements), genuine spirit of partnership, culture that promotes physician creativity, leadership, and long-term relationships between the hospital and the physician.

The ability to form a strong physician–physician, physician–investor, or physician–hospital partnership requires the partners to do the following:

- *Set a quality standard.* Although every physician must be clinically competent, the partners should be at the forefront of their respective fields and intolerant of less than high quality. Remember, quality is still the best measurement of success in most health care ventures.

- *Make entrepreneurial contributions to the partnership.* Every partner should participate in the entity's management, organization, and administrative structuring. Being a partner also means accepting the risks as well as the rewards. An individual who wants to practice good medicine for a guaranteed income should be an employee, not an owner or investor.
- *Make personal contributions to the partnership.* A partner must clearly add value to the entity by the work product and the output of that product. The result is increased revenues or other improvements within the practice. Ownership demands more time, energy, and commitment than one could expect from being an employee only.

The Political Fallout

Political fallout is possible after the formation of a partnership or diversified health care venture. For example, the surgeon who invests in the building and operation of an ASC may be alienated from the hospital (if not a partner in the venture) and other physicians. Certainly, this type of specialist depends on referrals for the continued viability of the practice, as well as the ASC. Such considerations should become part of the feasibility study, which is used to evaluate the proposed venture, in this case whether to build the ASC.

When considering a partnership or joint venture, assess what is best for the community as a whole and provides the best long-term results. A physician may benefit financially in the short run with an ancillary venture that, in the long run, may hurt the physician and the entire community if the new services take business from other caregivers in the area.

Political fallout may occur within the very group that is considering investing in the ancillary venture. For example, a multispecialty group may not have the backing of all of its partners for the investment in certain ancillary ventures. Also, the ASC that is to be constructed by a multispecialty group may not generate a great deal of interest among its primary care physicians. Thus, the overall initiative needs to be thoroughly discussed and agreed on before moving ahead, and all decisions should be made with the best interests of the entire group in mind.

Legal Constraints and Considerations

There are, of course, legal considerations relative to ancillary ventures and physician diversification. Both state and federal regulations require physicians and other health care entities to be in compliance relative to the delivery of services, regardless of the format under which they are practicing. Most regulations, whether they are federal anti-kickback statutes, Stark regulations, or other laws, focus on ensuring that the cost or delivery of care is not being impugned or in any way being taken advantage of due to the actions of the physicians.

The Stark regulations prohibit physicians from making referrals for certain designated health services (DHS) payable by Medicare to an entity with which they (or an immediate family member) have a financial relationship (ownership, investment, or compensation), unless an exception applies. DHS includes the following services and supplies:

- Clinical laboratory services
- Physician therapy, occupational therapy, and speech-language therapy
- Radiology and radiation therapy (now includes nuclear medicine)
- Durable medical equipment and supplies
- Parenteral-enteral nutrients
- Prosthetics
- Home health services
- Outpatient prescription drugs
- Inpatient and outpatient hospital services

The federal Stark law defines a group practice as a single legal entity in any organizational form recognized by the state in which the group is doing business. The group practice must have at least two physicians who are members of the group (whether employees, or direct or indirect owners). Stark defines a member of the group as a direct or indirect owner of a group practice (including physicians whose interests are held by their individual professional corporation or by another entity), a physician employee of the group practice, a locum tenens physician, or an on-call physician while the physician is providing on-call services for members of the practice. An independent contractor is not a member of the group. Each physician who is a *member of the group* must furnish substantially the full range of patient care services that the physician routinely furnishes, including medical care, consultation, diagnosis, and treatment, through the joint use of shared office space, facilities, equipment, and personnel.

Ancillary ventures, such as ASCs, must be structured so as to avoid raising legal and regulatory red flags. Therefore, it is critical to consult with a knowledgeable health care attorney who works full time on Stark and antitrust issues for advice on this very complex section of the law.

A number of states have enacted self-referral regulations, and legal due diligence should include review of the specific state provisions, which may include a broader list of DHSs. It should be noted that ASCs have been free from scrutiny under state self-referral laws. It is unlikely that an ASC venture that does not violate the Stark law would violate state law. However, state certificate-of-need (CON) requirements may exist. Currently, 14 states have no CON laws affecting hospitals or ASCs; the CON laws of 10 others do not apply to ASCs. If a CON is a consideration, the law often depends on the ASC's size, cost, structure, and location (see Figure 3-2).[2, 3] Any ancillary investment undertaken by physicians should be thoroughly reviewed by legal council to ensure legal compliance prior to the actual commencement of the project.

State	ASCs2	CON/No CON3	State	ASCs2	CON/No CON3
AK	9	CON	MT	15	CON
AL	36	CON	NC	69	CON
AR	63	No CON	ND	17	No CON
AZ	150	No CON	NE	44	No CON
CA	668	No CON	NH	21	CON
CO	101	No CON	NJ	201	No CON
CT	44	CON	NM	21	No CON
DC	4	CON	NV	50	CON
DE	25	CON	NY	87	CON
FL	358	No CON	OH	193	No CON
GA	253	CON	OK	51	No CON
HI	12	CON	OR	76	No CON
IA	25	CON	PA	221	No CON
ID	56	No CON	RI	7	CON
IL	120	CON	SC	62	CON
IN	125	No CON	SD	16	No CON
KS	63	No CON	TN	148	CON
KY	35	CON	TX	346	No CON
LA	72	No CON	UT	43	No CON
MA	56	CON	VA	48	CON
MD	357	CON	VT	1	CON
ME	17	CON	WA	221	CON
MI	80	CON	WI	58	No CON
MN	49	No CON	WV	11	CON
MO	97	No CON	WY	18	No CON
MS	64	CON			

CON: certificate of need

FIGURE 3-2 Ambulatory Service Center (ASC) Entrepreneurs

Conclusion

The concept of diversifying the traditional medical practice, as addressed in this chapter, is multifaceted and can occur in areas such as the business model as well as services the practice offers. The changing financial picture for physicians demands a response, a response that is proactive and resourceful. Some political fallout may occur within the medical community, however, as change always brings attention and often criticism. Further, physician diversification is at risk of scrutiny relative to Stark and antitrust issues, as noted. The physician practice should seek wise counsel in all matters regarding ancillary ventures.

Endnotes

1. Merriam-Webster Dictionary Online. Available at: http://www.merriam-webster.com/dictionary/retail. Accessed March 18, 2011.
2. Koenig L, Doherty J, Dreyfus J, Xanthopoulos J. An Analysis of Recent Growth of Ambulatory Surgical Centers: Final Report. Rockville, MD: KNG Health Consulting LLC, June 5, 2009. (Per the report, figures are based on 2007 Medicare data.) Available at www.ascassociation.org/study.pdf. Accessed March 16, 2011.
3. Cauchi R. Certificate of Need: State Health Laws and Programs. Washington, DC: National Council of State Legislatures. Available at www.ncsl.org/IssuesResearch/Health/CONCertificateofNeedStateLaws/tabid/14373/Default.aspx#2009. Updated April 30, 2009; material added January 28, 2010. Accessed March 16, 2011.

CHAPTER 4

Practice Buy-in/ Practice Buyout

OUTLINE

While there has been a dramatic increase in hospital employment of physicians over the past several years, the fact remains that many physicians (if not the majority) are still in private practice. Accordingly, practice buy-in and buyout scenarios remain a reality that must be addressed as physicians enter and exit ownership of the private medical practice. Potential practice purchasers and sellers must evaluate the various alternatives pertaining to the acquisition and divestiture of partnership interests. Often referred to as buying-in and buying-out of practice ownership, the process of acquisition and divestiture is critically important and has long-lasting effects on the practice's welfare and success. It requires thorough planning and design to fit the specific profile of the practice and its partners.

Equity Track Considerations

Most equity agreements are created during the formative stages of the practice. When a new practice is being formed, the existing partners must decide how the buy-sell process will work. This issue is less important when a solo practitioner starts a practice, unless the physician anticipates creating an avenue for adding new shareholders in the future. In addition, at certain points in time, physicians in a practice may choose to review and revise their equity agreements either to stay current with changes occurring in the marketplace or to respond to specific issues they are facing as a practice. These issues could include recruitment, a lack of ability to fund the current buyout plan, and a host of other potential concerns.

The practice's company agreement or operating agreement typically outlines the buy-sell process. As an example, consider the following language from a Texas medical practice's company agreement outlining how to add a new equity member.

2.4 Admission of New Equity Members.

(a) The Company may, from to time, admit as additional Equity Members individuals who are duly licensed to practice medicine in the State of Texas. The admission of an additional Equity Member and the terms and conditions of such admission shall require the approval of a Required Interest of the Equity Members. Unless otherwise determined by a Required Interest of the Equity Members, an individual will be admitted as an Equity Member only after being a Clinical Member for at least two years.

(b) Unless otherwise determined by a Required Interest of the Equity Members, a new Equity Member will be required to pay to the Company a buy-in amount equal to such new Equity Member's Interest multiplied by the excess of the fair market value of the fixed tangible assets of the Company as of the date such new

Equity Member is being admitted to the Company over any liabilities of the Company associated with such assets, all as determined in the reasonable discretion of a Required Interest of the Equity Members.

(c) No Person shall be admitted as an additional Equity Member unless such Person executes, acknowledges, and delivers to the Company such instruments as the Company may deem necessary or advisable to effect the admission of such Person as an additional Equity Member, including (without limitation) the written acceptance and adoption by such Person of the provisions of this Agreement and the entering into an Employment Agreement on terms mutually acceptable to such Person and the Company.

Also consider the following example as it relates to how the stock or equity interest of a practice will be valued.

(a) Upon any such sale of Stock by a Shareholder, the total value of the Corporation ("*Corporate Value*") shall be equal to the value of the practice's tangible assets. The Deceased, Disabled, Voluntarily Withdrawing, and Involuntarily Withdrawing Shareholder's Stock shall equal the Corporate Value multiplied by the Final Productivity Factor for the preceding twelve (12) months.

(b) In the event that the Shareholder has voluntarily resigned from his or employment by the Corporation upon less than three hundred sixty five (365) days prior written notice, the value shall be reduced as follows:

Days Notice of Resignation	Reduction to Value
0–60	30%
61–120	25%
121–180	20%
181–240	15%
241–300	10%
301–365	5%

(c) In the event that the Shareholder's employment terminated due to loss of medical license, exclusion from anticipation of the Medicare or Medicaid programs or loss of privileges at the Hospital, the value shall be reduced by 100%.

An issue that many practices face is that they may have formed their practice with a group of physicians many years ago. While they may have an equity agreement that specifically delineates how buy-in and buyout events will occur, they may simply not recall the intent. Also, they may disagree about what the language in the equity agreement really means, due to the time that has transpired between when they established the equity agreements and the first time they were actually effectuated. To avoid these types of situations, it is important for practices to revisit their operating agreements on a regular basis, every three to five years, to ensure that the information included is still consistent with their intent relative to how an equity event should be handled. Typically, such a process can be facilitated by a qualified health care attorney or health care consultant.

The Buy-In Process

The buy-in process usually involves an employed physician purchasing an equity interest in a practice. It could also entail an existing shareholder purchasing a larger amount of equity in the practice (although the latter rarely occurs).

Physician Eligibility for Buy-in

There is no rule for how practices must determine how or when a physician should become eligible to buy-in to a practice. As a result, an infinite number of methodologies exist. If all of the methodologies were consolidated into two specific approaches, they would likely reflect (1) years of service and (2) level of productivity.

Many practices simply state that after a certain number of years as an employed physician, physicians can become shareholders. The typical time requirements that exist within the industry are two to five years, with most practices using the lower end of the range. In some cases, practices develop a stair-step approach. Further, as more physicians consider becoming employed by hospitals instead of joining an existing private practice, the time requirement is often waived altogether, or limited to a shorter period of one year.

As an example, based on the excerpt provided earlier, after two years the physician may have the ability to become a "clinical member" of the practice and then, after a total of four years (two years after becoming a clinical member), the physician is granted full shareholder rights.

Table 4-1 outlines the key differences between a clinical member and a full shareholder. As a clinical member (after two years of employment), the physician gains some benefits of being a shareholder but only achieves full shareholder status after four years of employment. This stair-step approach is beneficial for practices that want to lengthen the partnership track period. It provides physicians with some benefits before becoming full shareholders, while retaining the incentive of ultimately achieving this objective.

Another method for determining qualification is to tie it to productivity. This assessment could be measured by various productivity metrics, most commonly cash collections or work relative value units (wRVU). In most instances, the practice establishes a threshold or

TABLE 4-1 Comparison of Clinical Member and Full Shareholder

	Clinical Member	Shareholder
Equity Interest	No	Yes
Voting Rights	No	Yes
Participate in Shareholder Income Distribution Plan	Yes	Yes
Share in Ancillary Profits	No	Yes

quota that buying-in physicians must achieve before being considered for shareholder status. In some cases, it may be tied to profitability. For example, buying-in physicians may be required to fully cover any financial loss that existed when they started and then generated a certain level of profit for the partners of the practice. Once these are fulfilled, physicians would be eligible to buy in. Some other examples of productivity qualifications are outlined as follows:

- An interventional cardiologist must achieve collections of $60,000 per month for four consecutive months.
- An internal medicine physician must achieve annual wRVUs equivalent to the 50th percentile, as outlined in the latest Physician Compensation and Production Survey from the Medical Group Management Association.
- Clinical member status will be granted after achieving the 50th percentile for collections, with full shareholder status being granted once 75th percentile collections are achieved.
- The physician must achieve collections that are consistent with the average collections or wRVUs for the other practice physicians.

Clearly, productivity thresholds can take many forms. The key is for the thresholds to be achievable by a reasonable physician over an appropriate period of time. Otherwise, it will likely create a disincentive, potentially causing physicians to leave the practice. Because private practices increasingly have to compete against hospitals for new physicians, there is a heightened sense of awareness relative to the reasonableness of the buy-in.

Establishing Practice Buy-in Value

The key question relative to the buy-in process is how much money is involved and how the buy-in amount is calculated. There are many possible ways to structure the purchase price and factors to which it can be tied. Due to the infinite number of possibilities, it is clearly impossible to outline them all. The following four alternatives are some of the key formula approaches used.

Alternative 1: Set Purchase Price

A common form of buy-in is a pre-established purchase price. In these instances, practices simply establish an amount that is associated with becoming a shareholder, and this figure applies to each new shareholder that is added. As an example, the purchase price could be $40,000. Thus, every new partner added is required to pay $40,000, which is then reallocated to the existing shareholders.

This approach is by far the simplest buy-in method, as it requires very little work when a buy-in event occurs. Further, it is very easy to inform new physicians of what will be required and to maintain consistency over time. It also limits the cost of the buy-in process. Because no formal valuation is needed, it often will require less work from legal counsel to accomplish.

Alternative 2: Tangible Assets

Another very common approach, which is not quite as simple and consistent as having a set purchase price, is determining the value based on the practice's tangible assets. While the practice owners may desire to inventory and assign a value to their assets themselves, or simply use the net book value of their assets, the best practice is to use an independent third party to perform a tangible asset valuation. This method is preferred because only looking at the net book value can undervalue certain assets if depreciation has been accelerated. Also, it can place no value on assets that may be fully depreciated but are still in full use. Thus, the best practice is to value using an in-place valuation methodology wherein the assets actually being used are considered and are valued based on their current status and functionality. In such cases, an independent valuation firm is hired to value the practice's tangible assets. That value is then used to assign a value to the interest a new physician is purchasing. The value is calculated on the basis of owned tangible assets, less any debt associated with those assets. Thus, any assets that are leased are excluded from the calculation. Consider the following example:

- Value assigned to tangible assets, less debt: $600,000
- Current shareholders: 10

The purchase price is calculated by determining the equity interest a new physician will purchase. As there will be 11 shareholders after the new physician purchases his or her equity interest, to obtain an equal interest, the physician will need to purchase 0.91% interest from each physician. Thus, the interest the new physician is purchasing is a 9.09%. When multiplied by the full practice tangible asset value, the buy-in interest totals $54,540.

Alternative 3: Full Practice Valuation

Another less common, but still often used method, of determining the purchase price of the practice is by performing a business valuation of the practice. This approach takes into consideration both the tangible and intangible assets associated with the practice. In many cases, adding intangible assets will result in a significantly higher value than the other methods outlined here.

The higher value may prove to be beneficial to the existing partners, as they are able to generate higher incomes when new physicians buy into the practice. However, this increased value can significantly inhibit recruitment, as physicians who are struggling to begin paying down their student loans do not want to be encumbered as well by a larger buy-in. This scenario is especially the case now, wherein a physician could become employed by a hospital, have little risk associated with managing a practice, and still generate a fair market value wage.

Alternative 4: Gifted Equity

While probably the least common of these four approaches, a potential method of assigning a purchase price is to not have a purchase price. The equity is essentially transferred without cost to the physician who is buying-in to the practice. In some cases, when the practice has been able to generate substantial profit from the employed physician's financial performance over the period of employment, such a process can make financial sense. In this approach, the shareholder physicians consider the profits reaped when the physician was an employed physician to be sufficient to cover any buy-in that would otherwise occur.

In other instances, for a variety of reasons, the shareholder physicians may choose to give equity to a buying-in physician even when it does not make total financial sense. This could be the result of a son joining a father's practice or a recruitment strategy to entice a prospective physician. Another reason may be that the physician has already been participating in the shareholder income distribution plan; therefore, very little would change if the physician were admitted as a partner.

Although from a financial perspective only limited benefits may be gained from such a method, operationally speaking it is clearly a very easy approach to effect.

In many situations, the purchase price is a blending of several of the alternative approaches. Consider the following examples:

- A physician is gifted a partial (less than equal) interest in the practice after a period of two years and then, once certain productivity thresholds are met, is able to purchase the remaining interest based on the value of the tangible assets.
- The purchase price is based on the lesser of the value of the tangible assets or $60,000.
- The value assigned to the entire practice, for purposes of calculating the purchase price for a single physician, will be based on the business valuation (both tangible and intangible assets) but will be no lower than $800,000 and no higher than $1 million.

Examples of Buy-in Alternatives

The method of purchase largely involves the (1) timing of the payment process and (2) treatment from a tax perspective. We will explore here several alternatives that typically exist relative to the timing of the payment.

Immediate Physician Buy-in

The first alternative is an up-front payment at the time the option to become a shareholder is available. In this scenario, regardless of the purchase price, physicians are required to submit the required funds in a lump sum at the onset of becoming a shareholder. Depending on the amount of the buy-in and the physicians' financial situation, this action could require physicians to borrow money to fund the buy-in. The borrowing could be in the form of a small-business loan from a local bank or a loan from the practice at a market rate of interest. Depending on the economic climate and/or the financial situation of the physicians (eg, level of student loans), it could be difficult for physicians to borrow the adequate level of funds, thus making becoming a shareholder challenging. Further, the practice may not have the funds to lend to physicians to fund the buy-in. If financing can be secured or if the buy-in amount is minimal so that funding is not necessary, an upfront payment is a legitimate alternative. In most situations, a buy-in that is based on a specific purchase price or only on the tangible assets would likely best effectuate this buy-in methodology.

Buy-in Over Several Years vs an Equity Track Formula

The second alternative, which is commonly used, is a payment over time. Thus, physicians may be allowed a period of 12 to 48 months to complete the buy-in process. This option tends to be more functional for new physicians than having to secure funds for an upfront payment. The key question with this approach is when physicians are granted full shareholder status in terms of voting rights, profit distributions, and the like. Full shareholder status can be granted at the onset of the buy-in process, incrementally, or at the conclusion of the buy-in process. Typically, an incremental approach is not taken because of the difficulty it creates in calculating physician compensation, etc. Thus, the key options are either at the inception or conclusion of the buy-in. The preferred method tends to be granting full shareholder status at the inception of the buy-in process.

Buy-in at the End of the Eligibility Period

A buy-in at the end of the eligibility period can be achieved by establishing the valuation total and a correlated buy-in amount at the beginning of the buy-in period or some time thereafter, including at the time of buy-in, which is at the end of the eligibility period. New physician partners do not have to pay any of this amount until the end of the equity track period, say three to five years. This arrangement allows physicians to accumulate excess earnings on their own and then contribute at the end of that period. Of course, the disadvantage is that the equity interest is purchased with after-income tax dollars. A slight advantage is the ability to accumulate excess monies and privately earn a return on that investment before having to contribute to the buy-in. The earnings on this corpus, however, are likely not sufficient to cover the tax liability that could otherwise have been avoided (by using pre-tax dollars).

Alternatively, the practice buy-in amount could be established at the beginning of the buy-in period but not paid until some years later. The physicians could, in theory, have a fixed buy-in price that is lower than the value of the practice would have dictated (ie, buy-in percentage interest times the valuation). In theory, the physicians would be paying for an equity interest, after an appreciation of value is actually realized over the total initially established. Obviously, this would be the case if the arrangement were established at the time of the buy-in some years after initial employment. However, it is still possible to accumulate wealth and contribute a portion of that wealth to the practice buy-in some years later.

Fund Receivables Through a Compensation Formula

In certain instances, the buying-in physicians must also purchase part of their accounts receivable. In essence, paying for receivables that the physicians initially built during the first few weeks or months of working at the practice. During that time, the physicians received full compensation. Although productivity may have been good, it was probably not enough to fund the direct and indirect overhead (including the compensation) of the employed physicians (now prospective partners). Consequently, when the partnership is achieved, the receivables that the new physicians are required to pay to offset those initially "fronted" dollars become part of the buy-in. In some cases, this initial loss could be covered through an income guarantee arrangement with a local hospital. In such a case, the physicians should not be required to repay this loss (ie, the value of the receivables).

Most buy-in plans quantify the amount of the receivables along with the value of the practice. As a consequence, the following components could total the buy-in amount:

- Accounts receivable
- Fixed assets
- Intangible asset value or goodwill

Most methodologies for funding these receivables via the buy-in payment allow the new physicians to pay the share of receivables in pre-tax dollars. Some methodologies require payment in after-tax dollars, which is unattractive. With the pre-tax approach, compensation is tied to a percentage of the average compensation of the senior physicians, which generally entails an increasing percentage over a specified period. An example follows:

Year 1: 65%

Year 2: 72%

Year 3: 80%

Year 4: 87%

Year 5: 94%

Over the five-year period, the physician's compensation gradually increases to that of the senior physicians. For this to be fair, productivity and resultant compensation under normal circumstances would need to be analyzed.

In Figure 4-1, the compensation earned by the new physician progressively increases with a portion reallocated to the senior physicians. The first two years of the reallocation process are strictly to fund the accounts receivable that the new physician had been fronted during that first year; $80,000 was deemed to be a reasonable total. In years 3 through 6, the final portion of the equity track period, the actual purchase of that equity interest was effectuated. This was done by reducing the compensation paid to the new physician and reallocating it in the form of compensation to the senior physician. Obviously, these dollars could have been left in the practice for future growth and expansion (ie, retained earnings). For purposes of this example, the totals were reallocated to the senior physician.

Because the new physician is not in a position to be paid as much income initially, the reduction in compensation is such that the new physician was still able to realize an increase in total compensation each year. For example, in year 3, when productivity would have justified

Buy-in Structure Assumptions

- Average compensation for "new" physician = $300,000
- Net asset value (excluding accounts receivable) = $25,000
- Physician given 1-year probationary period
- Probationary period followed by 5-year buy-in arrangement
- New physician attains full productivity at end of third year

Year	Compensation Earned by New Physician	Compensation Paid to New Physician	Reallocation to Senior Physician	Allocation to Funding Receivables
1	$230,000	$200,000	$ 0	$30,000
2	$280,000	$230,000	$ 0	$50,000
3	$300,000	$244,000	$ 56,000	$ 0
4	$300,000	$260,000	$ 40,000	$ 0
5	$300,000	$274,000	$ 26,000	$ 0
6	$300,000	$288,000	$ 12,000	$ 0
			$134,000	$80,000

FIGURE 4-1 Buy-in Example

$300,000, the actual compensation was $244,000, with the remaining $56,000 reallocated to the senior physician. In year 4, comparable totals resulted in compensation of $300,000 initially, but this was discounted to $260,000. However, it still resulted in an increase in total compensation compared to the prior year.

In the example of Figure 4-1, the total buy-in would have been completed with the $80,000 funding the receivables and the $134,000 being reallocated to the senior physician based on the tangible or intangible value of the equity portion being purchased by the new physician. The new physician completes this process without paying income taxes on the difference. If this practice is a subchapter S or corporation, partnership, or limited liability company in which the earnings are passed through, and if the new partner held a portion of that equity during the buy-in period, that portion of the earnings, unless reallocated to the senior physician in the form of compensation, would be passed through, and taxes would be paid by the new physician. If allocated strictly to the senior physician and paid to him or her in the form of compensation, the new physician would not have paid any taxes on those reallocated amounts. Rather the senior physician would be responsible for the income taxes on those earnings.

The other key discussion point relative to the method of purchase is how the buy-in is treated from a tax perspective. The buy-in can take the form of either a post-tax or a pretax transaction. In a post-tax transaction, the physician is paid a salary, less any applicable withholdings for taxes and benefits, and then pays the purchase price based on this "take-home pay." In a pretax transaction, the buy-in amount is withheld within the practice before the physician's compensation is calculated. Thus, the physician's gross compensation is less because the buy-in for that period has been withheld.

As an example, consider a physician with an annual salary of $400,000 and a buy-in amount of $60,000. For the year when the buy-in occurs, the physician's annual salary could be reduced to $340,000 to allow for the buy-in to occur. The $60,000 would then be redistributed to the shareholder physicians and included in their compensation.

The pretax method is favorable in that it reduces the buying-in physician's tax liability during the buy-in period because of the lower gross income. The pretax method makes little to no difference from the perspective of the partner physicians. The pretax method tends to be how most practices structure buy-in transactions.

Summary of Buy-In Process

This section outlined the key areas of focus in determining the buy-in process for employed physicians who are becoming shareholders. Although the process seems relatively simple, it can become complex very quickly because of the number of variables involved. The key is for the partners of the practice to decide on a method and consistently apply it, as needed. The method should be reconsidered on a regular basis to ensure that it is consistent with the direction of the practice and the health care industry as a whole. Consistent application is a key issue, as it would seem unfair to existing shareholders if the required purchase price is substantially lowered or the requirements to become a shareholder are softened soon after they complete the buy-in process.

Some of the key decisions that must be made relative to the buy-in process can be remembered easily as the four Ds:

- *Document* what the new physician must accomplish to be eligible for an equity interest.
- *Determine* the amount of equity the new physician is eligible to purchase.
- *Delineate* the method of purchasing the equity interest.
- *Define* the purchase price and the method for deriving it.

Finally, keep the process as simple as possible!

Practice Buyout

While the buy-in process occurs at the beginning of the physician's life cycle with the practice, the buyout process occurs at the end of this life cycle. A physician buyout occurs for several reasons, including retirement, death, disability, pursuit of other opportunities, and termination. In most cases, the buyout process is not impacted by the reason for the buyout, with the exception of termination. In some cases, if shareholders violate the terms of the employment agreement with the practice or the operating agreement, shareholders may forfeit their equity interest or receive a limited buyout. An example of this is provided in the sample buyout language near the beginning of this chapter. Other than these limited instances, the same buyout process will apply regardless of the reason.

As with the buy-in process, several factors must be considered when appropriately structuring how the buyout will occur. Some of these factors can be correlated with the buy-in process, while others are considerations that do not apply to the buy-in process. This section outlines the key areas of focus relative to structuring the most effective buyout for the practice, including alternatives, if applicable.

Determining the Buyout Amount

In many instances, practices will correlate the buy-in process and the buyout process. This is not to indicate that they specifically mirror each other, but they have similar characteristics. The prime example is in the amount of funds involved. A common term used within the health care industry in terms of structuring buy-sell agreements is "easy in/easy out." This term means that the buy-in process requires limited funds from the purchasing physicians, and the buyout process also entails limited funds in terms of the physicians' payout from the practice. Thus, from an economic standpoint, there is consistency between the two equity events.

Logically speaking, this makes sense because otherwise the transactions would be out of balance. For example, it would be unreasonable to have someone pay a substantial sum of money to purchase an equity interest in a practice only to have the operating agreement assign limited funds to the equity interest when the buyout occurs. This method would be akin to purchasing a share of stock at $1,000, knowing that in several years it could only be sold for $50. No one would be willing to make such an investment. However, ownership in a medical practice is different from purchasing stock in a publicly traded company, as most of the value associated with the medical practice is realized in the years of ownership through the compensation that is earned. Most practices pay out all funds as compensation. Very little value remains in the company, at least from a tangible perspective, hence the need for a minimal buyout.

Typically, the buy-in and buyout processes are correlated in terms of the funds involved. If limited funds are required to purchase an equity interest in the practice, physicians should expect a similar result when selling the equity interest. Similarly, if physicians pay a substantial amount for the equity interest, it is reasonable to expect a similar payout when leaving the practice.

The buyout amount can be calculated in a manner similar to the buy-in purchase. In fact, the purchase price can also establish the value for the buyout. This approach makes sense in that the two equity events are dealing with the same equity. However, the buy-in and buyout do not necessarily have to be correlated.

To reiterate some of the buy-in concepts and how they would apply to the buyout, this section outlines various alternatives.

Alternative 1: Established Value

Similar to the buy-in process, the value associated with the practice can be an established amount. Although it would make sense for the buy-in amount and the buyout amount to mirror each other, it is not always the case. For example, the buy-in could be established at $30,000 and the buyout could be established at $60,000. The opposite could be true as well.

Having an established amount has many benefits. It still recognizes some value associated with the equity interest, while maintaining it at a level that is functional for the practice from a cash flow perspective. Further, limited costs are incurred with each equity transaction, as there is less need for third-party appraisals of the business and legal costs.

Similar to the buy-in alternative, the accounts receivable are typically paid out to the physician in addition to any established purchase price.

Alternative 2: Tangible Assets

At the time of each equity event, the practice can have an independent appraiser place a value on the practice's tangible assets and let the assigned value establish the buyout amount. In this way, the share of the tangible assets and any collections generated from the physicians' existing accounts receivable balance would compose the buyout.

Alternative 3: Full Practice Valuation

The value also can be derived on the basis of the value associated with the entire practice, including both intangible and tangible assets.

As this method typically entails a higher valuation and resultant buyout amount, the practice must plan in advance for such an occurrence.

This alternative includes regularly setting aside funds, well before the equity event occurs, so that it can be funded through existing practice assets. Alternatively, an installment payment process should be instituted, wherein departing physicians are paid out over a period of years.

As in the buy-in process, limitations can be established relative to the buyout amount. For example, the buyout amount could be based on the lesser of the physicians' share of the value placed on the tangible assets or $80,000. Thus, it may be beneficial to have an independent valuator assess the value of the assets involved, but then there is a limitation on the maximum exposure of the practice from a payout standpoint.

Alternative 4: No Value Assigned

A final method of handling the buyout process is not to assign any value to the practice. Thus, physicians essentially leave with nothing. This option would make sense only if physicians did not pay anything for the equity interest in the buy-in process.

Considering how medical practices function, with literally all available cash being paid out as compensation to the physicians, this process makes sense in that all the value could be assumed to have been extracted while physicians were shareholders of the practice.

Even if no value is assigned to the practice, the physicians typically retain ownership of earned accounts receivable, which are paid out as they are collected. Thus, the physicians still receive some payout on leaving. Because the payout is funded from the accounts receivable, it has no negative impact on the cash flow of the practice.

Paying for the Buyout

A key issue with the buyout process is having the funds available to accomplish the transaction, especially when a substantial amount is involved. The majority of medical practices distribute all excess earnings, leaving very little compensation within the practice to fund replacement of equipment, expansion of services, and buyout of departing physicians. Thus, when physicians leaving the practice are eligible to receive a sizeable buyout, the practice must produce the needed funds. This method typically involves either reducing compensation for the existing physicians or borrowing money. Alternatively, the practice can plan for these buyout events well ahead of time by retaining funds in the corporation for this purpose.

Funding a buyout through debt is not a favorable idea, as the debt is not tied to any tangible asset, and the remaining physicians will need to pay off the debt over a period of years. An immediate reduction in compensation in the year of the physicians' departure is likely not tolerable either. Accordingly, an alternative approach must be considered, which typically involves the practice paying the buyout over a period of years.

For large buyouts, the payments can extend over a period of five years, whereas smaller buyouts can be limited to a period of 12 to 24 months. Funding the buyout over a period of years keeps the practice from having to borrow money and limits the reduction in the remaining physicians' compensation in a specific period. The physicians in the practice can then decide if interest is charged on any unpaid balance. For example, if the buyout is $50,000, the practice could pay interest on any unpaid balance at market rates.

Depending on how the buyout is structured, another means of funding the buyout is through the profits of newly added employed physicians. This approach typically applies only when retiring physicians are replaced with employed physicians. Once the employed physicians' productivity reaches the expected level (which should happen rather quickly, as the physicians are taking over an existing patient base), the retiring physicians are paid any profits generated by the newly employed physicians. This plan is in lieu of the profits being paid to the existing shareholders. Thus, from a cash flow perspective, the buyout has no impact on the existing shareholders, as it is contingent on the profits generated by the employed physicians. When this type of approach is applied, it tends to be for a limited period of time, typically 24 months. After that time, the profits generated by the employed physicians either increase those physicians' compensation or are paid to the existing shareholders.

Another key factor relative to the funding of a physician buyout pertains to the death of a physician. In this case, the buyout is funded through any life insurance proceeds the practice receives relative to policies held against the deceased. While not all practices hold life insurance policies on their physicians that are payable to the practice, this is key for situations in which a significant buyout exists, as it can cause potentially irreparable harm to the practice.

One aspect of the buyout process that should be considered is a potential waiting period. In many instances, it makes sense to require physicians to be shareholders of the practice for at least five years before a buyout can occur, particularly if the buyout is somewhat more lucrative than the buy-in. Further, practices often need to limit the number of physicians who can initiate a buyout during a given period. For example, the practice may limit equity events to one physician buyout in a 12- to 24-month period. This stipulation will allow the practice to better handle buyouts from a cash flow perspective.

Summary of the Buyout Process

The buyout process is somewhat less involved than the buy-in process, but it can still have significant financial ramifications on the practice's operations. Key decisions must be made as to how lucrative the buyout should be and how it will be funded. While a substantial buyout may sound appealing to individual physicians, it may not be so appealing when they experience a reduction in their compensation to fund a partner's buyout.

Although it is not required, the best practice is for the buy-in and the buyout to be economically consistent with one another. Thus, if limited funds are involved in the buy-in, the same should occur in the buyout. The opposite holds true as well: if a substantial buy-in is required, it is only reasonable to have a comparable buyout.

Physicians should not look at the buyout process as a means of funding their retirement. These funds should come through proper planning and savings throughout their career. Rather the buyout process should be viewed as a way to extract some, albeit mostly limited, value from the equity ownership within the practice.

Key Points to the Buy-in/Buyout Process

When buy-in and buyout agreements are created, the following key considerations should be a part of the process:

- Define the buy-in/buyout terms at the same time to ensure that they make sense when considered together.
- Define the terms for obtaining an equity interest at the onset of a potential shareholder's employment.
- Establish the eligibility requirements for becoming a shareholder.
- Establish the buy-in purchase price at an appropriate balance that is significant enough to be meaningful, but not such that it is unattractive.
- Structure the payment process associated with the buy-in so that it is functional for younger physicians who may also be managing substantial student loans.
- When possible, structure the buy-in to occur on a pretax basis.
- Avoid guarantees of partnership after certain criteria are met to ensure that some discretion can be applied by the existing shareholders.
- Consider recruitment, practice size, culture, philosophies, and economics as key factors when determining the appropriate buy-in formula.
- Real estate buy-ins should be handled separately from the practice buy-in. If possible, the real estate should be given a separate legal entity.
- From the onset of employment, ensure that prospective shareholders understand the governance and leadership terms and conditions that will apply as a shareholder.

- Allow existing owners to have some greater level of control from a governance and leadership perspective. Some powers may also be reserved for the original owners.
- Ensure that the prospective partner fits within the culture of the practice before an equity interest is offered. Compatible features should include a focus on attitude, collegiality, productivity, and expense savings/control.
- Limit the number of buyouts that can occur at the same time.
- To the extent possible, ensure that the buy-in and buyout are somewhat aligned.
- Ensure that the buyout method is such that the practice can fund it without a substantial impact on operations or the existing physicians' compensation.
- Structure the payout to occur over a period of years as opposed to a lump sum.
- Regularly review the practice's operating agreements to ensure that the buy-sell structure is consistent with the practice's intent and industry standards.

Attention to these factors will enable a good decision.

Conclusion

The focus of this chapter is two-fold. Practice owners should have a current plan in place that addresses the scope and the process of buying in to the practice. Likewise, a buyout process and protocol must also be planned and funded in advance to avoid tensions and conflict that are damaging to the practice. This chapter addresses each of these scenarios and points out the matters of primary importance and why and how they must be addressed.

2

PART TWO

Closing the Medical Practice

Chapters 5 and 6 address closing considerations for such reasons as retirement and transitioning of ownership. Here, the book examines components of the entity that will be affected by a practice closure, including operations, employees, patients, real estate and facility, and technology and information systems. Following a closing checklist will ensure that all matters will be properly handled in a timely manner, including attention to cash equivalents, and other assets, accounts receivables, accounts payables, legal entity termination, and transitioning.

CHAPTER 5

Considerations for Selling or Closing a Practice

OUTLINE

I. Introduction
II. Practice Sales
III. Closing a Practice for Personal Reasons
IV. Operational Considerations Relative to Closure
    A. Collecting Accounts Receivable
    B. Settling Accounts Payable
    C. Allowing Access to Medical Records
    D. Resolving Unpaid Claims
    E. Managing the Revenue Cycle
    F. Controlling Expenses
V. Employee Considerations Relative to Closure
    A. Employment
    B. Benefits
VI. Physician Responsibility to Patients
    A. Patient Notification Requirements
    B. Transitioning Patients and Ownership
VII. Real-Estate, Facility, and Market Value Considerations
    A. Understanding the Marketplace
VIII. Technology and Information Systems Considerations
    A. Security
    B. Record Retention and Patient Access
    C. Value of Electronic Health Record Technology
IX. Professional Liability and Tail Coverage
X. Final Liquidation of Assets and Closure
XI. Conclusion

The sale or closure of a medical practice is a complicated matter requiring thoughtful consideration on many levels. An owner can sell a practice based on numerous factors, and the sale can be made to several entities. Issues other than a desire to sell can generate a practice closure; namely, retirement, health or disability, or other personal reasons.

This chapter addresses the important decisions that a physician owner must make and actions to take in the process of sale or closure of a medical practice. The owner has responsibilities from several perspectives, including as a business operator and manager, as an employer to employees, as a licensed physician to patients, as a facility owner, and as an insured individual who must maintain liability protection.

Practice Sales

Physicians may sell their practice to other physicians or to a limited selection of other entities. The sale of practices varies from community to community and from specialty to specialty. Also, states vary in their requirements for broker licensing. If practice owners engage brokers or consultants to assist in the sale, the owners should check with the state to determine if licensure is required, and then verify the agents' credentials. Physician sellers should request a copy of the law and consultants' credentials and should not rely on a verbal response, as laws change and interpretations may vary. Licensed consultants and brokers are required to provide a copy of their license number.

When physicians sell to partners in an existing practice, it is important for their personal attorneys to review carefully the arrangements of the agreement with the partners and to advise on any concerns.

Closing a Practice for Personal Reasons

Physicians may decide to close a practice for various personal reasons, such as retirement, disability or other health-related issues, or to pursue another career. Closing a medical practice for personal reasons requires thought and preparation. In the case of planning for retirement, ideally, preparation should begin as long as three years or more in advance of retirement. This forethought allows for time to sell or rent the practice to another physician and inform patients and insurers. Owners should also contact the state medical board if the intent is to forgo renewing their medical license and obtain rules regarding notification of patients and transfer of medical records. Also, the local Drug Enforcement Administration (DEA) office should be notified if controlled substances are on the premises so that the agency can remove them safely, and the malpractice carrier needs notification to clarify tail coverage requirements.

To prevent fraud, retiring physicians also will have to surrender all prescription pads and documents that have a medical license number, name, and office address printed on them.

Many physicians hire associate physicians a few years prior to retirement and sell them their medical practice. This plan helps patients form solid relationships with new physicians so they stay in the practice after retiring physicians leave.[1] Renting the practice facility to an associate or another physician is another option to selling. This approach allows for additional income until owners are ready to sell. Closing a practice outright is not recommended, as the income from the sale may be necessary to pay any outstanding debts, assuring a comfortable retirement.

Regardless of the reason for closure, careful attention to many details must occur. Figure 5-1 is a checklist and timetable for preparing for a practice closing.

Time Period	Assignment	Assigned To	Date Completed
2 years prior	Reduce accounts receivable through improved collection techniques		
	Review and establish retirement objectives and financial plans		
	Begin searching for a buyer		
1 year prior	Review the office lease termination clause		
	Contact attorney and accountant		
	Seek legal advice on state laws for closure or transfer		
	Review equipment leases for termination		
	Escalate the collection process on accounts receivable		
6 months prior	Obtain a copy of the state's medical record laws and rules		
	Contact attorney and/or accountant about retention of billing, bank, employment, tax and legal records		
	Review termination clause in all payer contracts		
	Notify employees of plans to close		
	Decide on dispersal and/or storage of patient medical records		

FIGURE 5-1 Closing Checklist (*continues*)

Time Period	Assignment	Assigned To	Date Completed
	Set up a budget for office closure expenses: labor, equipment and supplies, utilities, alternative administrative space, moving expenses, and storage space		
	Plan for disposition of equipment, furniture, supplies		
3 months prior	Notify active patients in writing		
	Place an advertisement in local newspaper		
	Decide how to handle accounts receivable—outside agency or current employees		
	Start closing out accounts receivable		
	Notify local Drug Enforcement Administration (DEA) for approved method of drug disposal		
	Notify professional liability carrier of intent to close the practice and physician's plans for treating patients in another capacity		
	Notify creditors of closure in writing		
	Keep copies of all notifications		
1 month prior	Miscellaneous notifications to utility companies, telephone, answering service, janitorial service, linen service, landscaping, vending machines, etc		
	File a change of address with postal service		
	Cancel all periodicals		
	Notify the Board of Medical Examiners		
	Notify professional organizations (state medical society, AMA, specialty society)		
	Notify local hospital answering service about patient coverage		
Upon Closing	Destroy remaining prescription pads		
	Keep narcotics ledger as required by DEA		
	Dispose of all drugs per DEA instructions		
	Forward mail		
	Record telephone message for patients		

FIGURE 5-1 Closing Checklist (*continued*)

Operational Considerations Relative to Closure

Many details must be addressed to settle the finances of the practice, terminate the legal entity, dispose of assets, and inform necessary individuals and parties that the practice is closing. Legal guidance is important with many of these issues, and a paid consultant to manage some or all of these issues may be money well spent to ease the burden of practice closure, especially if a practice manager is not employed or does not remain available.

Collecting accounts receivable, settling accounts payable, allowing access to patient records, resolving unpaid claims, managing the revenue cycle, complying with regulatory requirements, controlling expenses, and dissolving the legal entity are discussed in the following sections.

Collecting Accounts Receivable

Develop a plan to collect accounts receivable. The decision to send accounts to collection should be balanced against both the cost of these actions and the ill will they generate; often, payment plans can be negotiated with patients who have outstanding debt to the practice. It will be necessary to write off some accounts as bad debt.

Settling Accounts Payable

When informing vendors, lessors, utility companies, and others listed in Figure 5-2, ask for invoices that settle accounts to be marked *Final Bill* by the issuer.

Allowing Access to Medical Records

Regardless of whether the physician permanently closes, rents the practice facility, or sells the practice, patient records must be available to patients. Under federal law, a physician must keep patient medical records at least seven years from the date of the last medical service for which there is a medical record entry. While individual states generally govern how long medical records are to be retained, **Health Insurance Portability and Accountability Act (HIPPS)** rules require a Medicare fee-for-service provider to retain required documentation for six years from the date of its creation or the date when it last was in effect, whichever is later.

Centers for Medicare and Medicaid Services (CMS) require that providers submitting cost reports retain all patient records for at least five years after the closure of the cost report. If the sellers are Medicare managed care program providers, CMS requires that patient records be retained for 10 years.

Contact/Action	√	Notes
(State) board of medical practice		
Federal Drug Enforcement Administration		
(State) Office of Controlled Substances (Controlled Substances Act) license		
Hospital(s) re: privileges		
Outpatient/nursing home facilities		
Insurance carriers		
Malpractice carrier		
Office leasing/management		
Bank/financial institutions		
US Postal Service		
Utility companies		
Computer IT /Internet		
Software vendor		
Computer hardware		
Office/medical vendors		
Professional organizations		
News/magazine subscriptions		
(State) Medical Society		
(location of medical records)		
Others:		

FIGURE 5-2 Offices and People Needing Notification of Office Closing

A minor patient's medical record is retained until a year after the patient reaches age 18 years, even if that period is longer than seven years. State laws also have an impact on medical records retention and availability to patients.

If owners are renting the facility or selling the practice, they should offer to send records to new physicians, if patients want to leave their practice for another. (Figure 5-3 is a sample Release of Records form for patients.) Patients can also elect to see the physicians who take over your office. Patient records can be transferred to these new physicians. Patients may also obtain their records under Health Insurance Portability and Accountability Act (HIPAA) guidelines. Contact the state's medical board for record-keeping and notification procedures and additional guidance.

Resolving Unpaid Claims

It is also important that physicians make every effort to submit claims for payment as soon as possible after the delivery of service so that most claims are paid prior to the closing of the practice. However, even with careful planning and prompt billing, it is likely that some unpaid claims remain at the time the practice closes. It will be necessary to have someone available to accept, record, and deposit payments received after the official closing of the practice. Thus, physicians should keep open the practice's bank account well past the closing date. Physicians could consider turning claims over to a reputable collections agency if they remain unpaid after a period of three or four months has elapsed since the first bill was sent.

Managing the Revenue Cycle

In the years and months preceding the sale or closure of a medical practice, it is critical to manage the revenue cycle to achieve the highest level of financial performance. Proper management and supervision of the revenue cycle includes the internal revenue cycle as well as the external revenue cycle. Figure 1-2 identifies the key components of both the internal and external revenue cycles. The practice that properly manages each of these areas of operation, all of which contribute to an effective and efficient payment strategy, will be better prepared when the practice is sold. Moreover, in all likelihood, it will enhance its value.

Influences on the external revenue cycle require attention, including managed care implications and governmental regulations. Compliance with regulatory rules (including HIPAA, the Occupational Safety and Health Administration [OSHA], Medicare, state medical board guidelines, and the Food and Drug Administration [FDA]), which requires significant effort, is a major factor for medical practices. All efforts to adhere to requirements must continue during the period preceding the sale or closure of the practice.

Request for Records Release

Physician's Name: ______________________________

Street Address: ______________________________

City: ____________________ State: ________ Zip: ____________

The following individual has asked us to request that his/her medical records be released and forwarded to the above listed office:

Patient Name: ______________________________

Birth date: ____________________ Social Security Number: ____________

Please be sure to include x-ray films and reports.

Thank you for expediting this request. Please send these records to our office address shown above.

Patient Authorization

I hereby authorize the release of all medical records to ____________________. I wish for them to be forwarded as soon as possible.

Please provide me with a copy of the medical records. I understand I will be charged a fee of $___ for this service.

Patient's Signature: ____________________ Date: ____________
(parent or guardian if patient is a minor)

Patient's Address: ______________________________

City: ____________________ State: ________ Zip: ____________

Signature of Witness: ____________________ Date: ____________

FIGURE 5-3 Request for Release of Medical Records

Controlling Expenses

As discussed in Chapter 1, expense controls fall into two categories: (1) internal controls that safeguard the handling of cash, and (2) controls that guard the way funds are expended. Practices should have internal controls in place to prevent or minimize the risk of embezzlement or other office thievery or misuse. When initiated, internal controls will reduce the chance for illicit activities to occur. In general, medical practices use a cash-based accounting method. It is imperative to ensure that all fees are billed, after applying discounts and contractual allowances, and collected.

Employee Considerations Relative to Closure

Employers have certain responsibilities to their employees during a closure or sale of a practice. These relate to actual employment, as well as to the way that benefits are handled. Physician owners have an obligation to address these issues professionally and to be in compliance with state and federal employment laws.

Employment

Employee hiring and firing must be handled with extreme caution by buyers and sellers. From the sellers' perspective, the policy should be to officially terminate each employee. Termination pay, severance pay, accrued vacation, accrued sick leave, as well as other issues must be reconciled between the two parties and addressed with the employees.

Benefits

Not all benefits result in a liability to sellers of the practice. For example, assuming that sellers recognize accrued vacation as a liability, the sellers and buyers can negotiate this point for assumption of liability. If buyers agree to recognize accrued vacation in time off during the first year of ownership, the two parties may resolve this circumstance accordingly. In contrast, buyers may not want to extend paid vacation leave, under the assumption that employees under the new employment relationship have not earned that vacation. Terminated employees may warrant a cash payment by the sellers for the accrued vacation. These matters must be discussed, outlined, and resolved prior to the announcement of sale. Employees are entitled to clear communication of benefits so they know exactly how they are affected.

Responsibility for health insurance benefits must transfer to the new owners. If the practice employs 20 or more persons, the new owners are subject to a continuation of coverage under the provisions of the Consolidated Omnibus Budget Reconciliation Act (COBRA) regulations. This potentially entails an additional cost to the employees because COBRA requires them to pay the full premium for health insurance if they continue under the health plan.

Other benefits must be effectively transitioned from the old practice to the new. Sick leave, disability insurance, retirement benefits, and life insurance must be converted. When the practice is acquired, whether it includes the actual legal entity or assets only, the new owners will establish their own benefits package and are not required to offer or assume the prior owners' package. Employees can benefit from the sale if the new owners offer an improved benefit package; this commonly occurs when physician owners sell to a larger health system (eg, a hospital, private corporation) with a comprehensive benefits plan.

Physician Responsibility to Patients

Physicians who close their offices have legal, ethical, and practical obligations to their patients. It is the physicians' responsibility to protect the patients' health information while at the same time ensuring its availability for continuity of care. To avoid any possibility of abandonment (the unilateral termination of the physician/patient relationship by the physician without the patient's knowledge or notification and without giving the patient sufficient opportunity to secure the services of another physician), patients should be notified of the practice closing by letter. If the practice is being sold to another physician, the patients should be notified of the name and address of the physician who is buying the practice. Various state laws, medical board regulations, and medical malpractice company guidelines have an impact on these obligations.

Patient Notification Requirements

Posting a small handwritten sign in the office or informing patients by word of mouth is not sufficient notification of a practice closure. A letter should be sent to all established patients *(those who have received professional services within the past three years from exiting physicians or from other physicians of the same specialty belonging to the same group practice)* at least 60 to 90 days in advance of closure. Sample letters are provided in Figures 5-4, 5-5, and 5-6. The notification letter should include the following information and forms:

- When the practice will be closing
- The reason for closing
- Notification of where the records will be stored and how to access them
- The need for the patient's written authorization to transfer medical records, and a request that written authorizations be returned by a specified date
- An authorization form for the patient to complete and return
- Encouragement for patients to begin looking for a new physician immediately
- A thank you for the opportunity to have been their physician

As also stated in Chapter 6, letters to patients do not need to be sent by certified or registered mail. The only requirement is to make a reasonable attempt to notify patients, so regular mail is sufficient. However, with particularly high-risk patients, certified or registered mail with a requested return receipt might be prudent. Place a copy of the notification letter in each patient's chart as well as any returned letters, with the associated envelopes, in the appropriate patients' charts. Again, there are state-specific requirements regarding patient notification. Check with the state medical licensure board or malpractice insurer for the requirements in your state.

The list in Figure 5-2 will help to identify offices and people with whom the practice does business and that need to be notified about the closing of the office. There may be additional contacts, but this list provides a good starting place.

Transitioning Patients and Ownership

Think about the impact on patients when the decision is made to sell a medical practice, particularly those with whom long-term patient-physician relationships have been formed. Patients see physicians as confidants and treat them with respect. It can be upsetting when their physicians leave or new physicians join the practice. Although networking makes it impossible to keep the sale confidential, patients need official notification when a change in medical practice ownership occurs. An exception exists when no changes are made in the physician staff (ie, when a hospital system purchases a practice). In this event, it is actually preferable for the transition to be as seamless as possible. If the community becomes aware of the sale, a letter of reassurance to all patients is vitally necessary.

Date:

Dear Mr/Mrs/Ms:

Please be advised that because of my (retirement/reasons of health/etc). I am discontinuing the practice of medicine as of (date). I shall not be able to provide services to you after that date.

I suggest that you arrange to identify another physician to provide your health care. If you are not acquainted with another physician, I suggest that you contact a hospital physician referral service. I shall make your medical records available to the physician you designate, or you can request a copy of your medical records [for a fee]. Since the records of your care are confidential, I shall require your written authorization to make them available to another physician. I am including an authorization form with this letter. Please complete the form and return it to me. I am sorry that I cannot continue as your physician. I extend to you my best wishes for your future health and happiness.

Yours very truly,

Name, (M.D./D.O.)

FIGURE 5-4 Letter for Physicians Discontinuing Practice

Date:

Dear Patients:

I am writing this letter to you with mixed emotions. I am now announcing my decision to sell my practice, effective (date) _________. This has not been an easy decision for me to make. Caring for my patients has been a great source of satisfaction and pleasure these past years.

I am anxious that you continue to receive quality medical care. I am, therefore, pleased to announce that as of (date)_________, Dr. (full name) _________ will be taking over my practice. Dr. (name) _________ is a graduate of (name of medical school) _________. He/She served his/her internship at (name of hospital) _________ in (location) _________, and he/she completed his/her residency in (specialty)_________ at (name of institution) _________. It is reassuring to me to be able to leave my patients in the hands of such a well-trained physician.

Of course, you are free to seek care elsewhere, if you wish; if so, please begin looking for another doctor as soon as possible. If you do not know where to begin, I suggest you contact your insurance company for a referral from their provider directory. If you do not have insurance, you may contact your local hospital's physician referral service. In any event, be sure to check with your insurer or managed care organization to verify that the services of the physician or physicians you are considering selecting are covered by your health plan. In the event a medical emergency arises in the interim, please remember that assistance is always available from the Emergency Department of your local hospital.

The contents of your medical chart are confidential and can be transferred to another doctor only with your permission. If you plan to see a physician other than Dr. (name)_________, please sign the enclosed authorization form and return it to my office as soon as possible. You may also obtain a copy of your records [for a fee]. Your records will continue to be on file in my former office. If you elect to be treated by Dr. (name)_________, you should sign an authorization form on or before your next visit to the office to release your records to his/her files.

I have valued my relationship with you, my patients, more than I can express in words. I thank you for your many years of loyalty and friendship. My staff and I extend our best wishes for your future health and happiness.

Sincerely,

_________, M.D./D.O.

FIGURE 5-5 Letter for Physicians Selling to Other Physicians

Date:

Dear Patients:

I am writing this letter to you with mixed emotions. I am now announcing my retirement from active practice, effective (date) _________. This has not been an easy decision for me to make. Caring for my patients has been a great source of satisfaction and pleasure these past years.

I am anxious that you continue to receive quality medical care. I'm therefore pleased to announce that as of (date)_________, Dr. (full name) _________ will be taking over my practice. Dr. (name) _________ is a graduate of (name of medical school) _________. He/She served his internship at (name of hospital) _________ in (location) _________, and he/she completed his/her residency in (specialty)_________ at (name of institution) _________. It's reassuring to me to be able to leave my patients in the hands of such a well-trained physician.

Of course, you're free to seek care elsewhere if you wish; if so, please begin looking for another doctor as soon as possible. If you don't know where to begin, I suggest you contact your insurance company for a referral from their provider directory. If you do not have insurance, you may contact your local hospital's physician referral service. In any event, be sure to check with your insurer or managed care organization to verify that the services of the physician or physicians you are considering selecting are covered by your health plan. In the event a medical emergency arises in the interim, please remember that assistance is always available from the Emergency Department of your local hospital.

The contents of your medical chart are confidential and can be transferred to another doctor only with your permission. If you plan to see a physician other than Dr. (name)_________, please sign the enclosed authorization form and return it to my office as soon as possible. You may also obtain a copy of your records [for a fee]. Your records will continue to be on file in my former office. If you elect to be treated by Dr. (name)_________, you should sign an authorization form on or before your next visit to the office to release your records to his/her files. I have valued my relationship with you, my patients, more than I can express in words. I thank you for your many years of loyalty and friendship. My staff and I extend our best wishes for your future health and happiness.

Sincerely,

_________, M.D./D.O.

FIGURE 5-6 Letter for Physicians Retiring and Selling to Other Physicians

Real Estate, Facility, and Market Value Considerations

When considering selling the practice and becoming an employee, physicians who own the building in which the practice resides must decide whether to sell the building along with the practice. Usually, physician sellers have accumulated nearly all of the equity in the building and have very little, if any, remaining debt. Further, they have exhausted most of the depreciable basis of the building, leaving virtually no cost basis in the structure. After selling the practice and the building, most of the proceeds of the sale of the building (which is a separate transaction from the practice) result in taxable gain. Although this taxable gain is subject to lower than ordinary income capital gains rates, it is still fully taxable. A significant tax burden can result when this occurs simultaneously with the sale of the practice.

Another choice during transition of ownership may be to retain the building, sell the practice, and lease the building to the new owners. This plan protects the equity and holds no further tax implications other than taxation of the ordinary income received from leasing the building. This arrangement would provide the building owners with additional revenue.

Many actions can be taken to prepare for the sale of the practice. Of course, the goal of any sale is to attain maximum value, whether the sellers continue as employees after the sale or completely sell and leave that practice. The initial basis for negotiating the sales price is the valuation. However, before the appraiser performs the valuation (or perhaps during its completion), the current owners can enhance the practice's value.

Understanding the Marketplace

The first step is to analyze the practice's market position by examining the practice's relationship to national, regional, and local economies. Also, review its position within the specific profession. Sources of information include the following:

- Market analysis
- Feasibility study
- Study of principles that influence values (eg, supply and demand, competition, changing conditions)

An understanding of the local marketplace is important to prospective sellers. Important components must be considered, and a discussion of each follows. The professional medical practice is a business with competitors nearby. It is conceivable (and likely) that the practice being sold is similar to other practices in a local area. This varies, however, with population centers. For example, in rural areas where medical practices are scarce, competition is minimal. Demand increases value in areas where limited or no competition exists.

Payer mix significantly influences the assessment of market conditions of the practice. If the patient population is covered by Medicare and Medicaid, expect significant discounting of fees (which may be offset by a higher volume of patients). In an environment in which managed care dominates, fees are either discounted or capitated. In a more traditional, fee-for-service patient population, the fee structure will yield a more lucrative practice and result in a higher value and sales price.

Economic conditions, including general health care supply and demand, affect practice values and, ultimately, the sales price. Trends in population, employment, and income that are continually changing influence economic stability. Economic conditions also affect a practice's ability to expand; likewise, they affect the sellers' ability to obtain an acceptable sales price.

Research current trends by asking the following questions: Is the practice in a growing community? Are people leaving the area? What is the local industry and is it growing? What are the ages of the residents? What is the unemployment rate? How many new jobs were created in the last year? These indicators influence general economic conditions and ultimately the sale of the practice.

The economic principle of supply and demand applies here as well. The value of a practice is influenced by the number of buyers available compared with the number of practices for sale. Evaluate how many similar practices are on the market and if the demand for them is declining. If it is a buyer's market, the sales price of that practice will be reduced. Conversely, if demand for a certain type of specialty practice increases and the supply remains constant (ie, no new practices of this type are opening), the price for that specialty practice should increase.

In general, the demand for established practices in most areas of the country has grown rapidly as health care continues to transition. Due to increased costs, the number of group practices is on the rise, and solo practices are diminishing in quantity. Physicians entering private practice are either purchasing existing businesses from their retiring colleagues, moving, or shifting to employed (salaried) positions. In addition, practices are operated as competitive businesses.

When making an offer on an existing practice, prospective purchasers should base the offer on recent selling prices of comparable practices and on the expected return on investment. From the sellers' view, acceptance of an offer depends on the minimum amount that buyers could purchase an equally desirable practice and the least amount the seller is willing to accept for that practice. This second point is influenced by the acceptable options available if the seller refuses to sell.

Selling a medical practice is an emotional undertaking. Practicing medicine is a way of life, and most physicians are profoundly dedicated to their profession and their patients. Although emotion does not alter the objective value of the practice, it does affect the owners' perception of its value (see Chapter 1).

Social, political, legal, and governmental factors also influence the value of a practice. Local and national statutes along with professional ethics regulate the organization of a medical practice and restrict the ownership to licensed practitioners. These elements significantly limit the marketplace.

Chapter 7, the Concepts of Value, and Chapter 8, the Valuation Process, provide additional information on preparing a practice for a valuation.

Technology and Information Systems Considerations

Physicians with electronic health record (EHR) systems have certain responsibilities for those records, including compliance with HIPAA security rules and medical record retention and patient access. In addition, the value of technology owned by the practice is also a point of debate. This section addresses these areas of concern.

Security

The HIPAA Security Rule applies to all individually identifiable health information in electronic format. Physicians must assess risks and vulnerabilities and protect the security and integrity of the health care record against threats. Physicians may use a variety of means, including firewalls, passwords, and encryption, to ensure that electronic medical records are secure.

Record Retention and Patient Access

Physicians who have electronic rather than paper medical records must still comply with the laws regarding medical record retention and patient access, which may require retention for varying time periods after the close of the practice. Ultimately, physicians must ensure that computerized medical data are permanently destroyed. Using the standard "delete" method generally results in deletion of the file name, while leaving recoverable data. Total destruction can be achieved by overwriting the information on the computer and destroying back-up tapes or by "wiping" the drive with a computer program that is designed to eliminate all specified data.

Value of Electronic Health Record Technology

Often the value of an EHR system can be an issue of dispute. While it decreases in value, similar to other equipment in the practice, it is slightly different. A good EHR system that can be integrated into a new system or that can be upgraded to work with a different system should be worth more as part of the sale. While it may be an older system, the EHR contains patient data, and its transfer from an existing system would decrease the cost of reentering the information into a new system.

Professional Liability and Tail Coverage

Physicians must work closely with their practice's malpractice insurance company when closing a practice to ensure appropriate coverage for potential claims that may arise after the discontinuation of patient care. Generally, malpractice policies are written on either "an occurrence" or a "claims-made" basis. Physicians must check with their agent if they are not sure which type of policy they have.

A claims-made policy only covers claims that take place and are reported to the insurer during the policy period. In general, physicians must purchase an extended reporting endorsement known as "tail insurance" for protection after termination of a claims-made policy. Most claims-made policies include a guaranteed right to purchase tail coverage within a specified time period. "Tail insurance" should be maintained until all statutes of limitation have run out.

An occurrence policy covers claims that arise out of incidents that occur during the policy period irrespective of when the claim is reported or filed. Thus, a physician with occurrence coverage will not require tail coverage. Physicians who change from a claims-made policy to an occurrence policy must obtain "nose," "tail," or prior-acts coverage to cover claims prior to the effective date of the occurrence policy.

Prior acts or nose coverage is essentially the same as tail coverage, but is generally acquired through a new insurer. When the extended reporting endorsement is purchased from the new insurance company (policy or carrier that physician is acquiring or joining), it is nose coverage. When the extended reporting endorsement is purchased from the insurance carrier or policy the physician is leaving, it is known as tail insurance.

Final Liquidation of Assets and Closure

Physicians leaving a practice must consider how to dispose of the physical assets of the practice, including the real estate, equipment, stocks of medications, and supplies. Disposal of medications are covered by the Secure and Responsible Drug Disposal Act of 2010 and may also be governed by state law, which should be consulted before actions are taken. Leases for space and equipment need to be terminated properly in writing to protect physician sellers from later claims that contracts were unilaterally broken. When assets are owned by the practice that is closing, they can be sold, auctioned, or donated. Often the practice's accountant can recommend the most financially advantageous option, if this is a consideration.

Conclusion

Closing a medical practice demands serious contemplation over an extended period to allow ample time to address all the considerations and complete the entire continuum of work. This includes due diligence, valuation, marketing, actual identification of a potential buyer through the agreement process, and, ultimately, the dissolution and transitioning processes. Physicians deserve to receive fair value for the hard work and dedication that have gone into building a strong patient base and revenue stream.

To attain the highest possible valuation, the practice must be open to review, due diligence, and scrutiny by prospective purchasers. It is important to obtain professional services from outside consultants who are savvy in the process of selling the medical practice and understand the valuation process. Both buyers and sellers should fully document all details of the purchase and sales agreement.

Sellers of the practice should understand and identify the reasons for selling. Moreover, they must prepare the practice for sale, develop market strategies to receive the true value, obtain an acceptable valuation of the practice, and seek assistance from professionals. Proper planning will result in substantiated legal documentation. The matters of dissolution of the practice, if applicable, should also be considered (see Chapter 6). Finally, an effective transitioning process from the sellers to the new owners is essential. The significance of this undertaking cannot be overstated.

Endnote

1. Jones J. Guidelines for Closing a Medical Practice. Bellevue, WA: eHow. http://www.ehow.com/way_5480476_guidelines-closing-medical-practice.html. Accessed May 18, 2011.

CHAPTER 6 Dissolution Considerations

OUTLINE

I. Introduction
II. Closing Checklist
III. Cash Equivalents and Other Assets
IV. Accounts Receivable
V. Accounts Payable
VI. Tax Considerations
  A. Property Taxes
  B. Payroll Taxes
  C. Income Taxes
VII. Legal Entity Termination
VIII. Transitioning to New Owners
  A. Patients
  B. Managed Care Organizations
  C. Personnel
  D. Employee Hiring and Firing
  E. Record Keeping
  F. Health Insurance Benefits
  G. Other Benefits
IX. The Phase-out Agreement
X. Conclusion

Once you have a contract for the sale of the practice, that business entity will be dissolved. There are many components of a dissolution that must be addressed to ensure sellers do not lose money. Many physicians incorporate a dissolution plan into the partnership agreement that is created when the business is started. In the absence of such an agreement, physicians can create a dissolution agreement any time prior to the planned closure of the practice to address the broader legal elements of the dissolution. The sale typically includes very specific assets of the medical practice. Tangible and intangible assets outside of the sale must be distributed prior to formal dissolution of the legal entity covering the practice, as discussed in Chapters 1 and 5. An attorney should be retained to guide the dissolution process and to help ensure legal and federal compliance of the transaction

Closing Checklist

Regardless of the reason for closing the practice, eg, retiring, relocating, selling, or closing, adequate planning can ease the transition for everyone involved. Using a simple checklist to guide each step in the process helps to ensure (refer to Figure 5-1) that all the appropriate steps have been taken in an orderly fashion, increases the efficiency of the process, and helps to ease the anxiety of such an undertaking. If closing the practice has been part of a long-term plan to sell, it is even more important to recognize ways to increase the value of the practice, well in advance of the transaction. Although this list is not exhaustive, it provides a framework for considerations and will help to initiate additional thoughts and plans around the closure of the practice.

Cash Equivalents and Other Assets

As discussed in Chapter 1, the allocation and distribution of cash equivalents and other assets must be defined before dissolving the practice. These decisions must be made before dissolving the practice, because the assets could be dispersed in different ways, depending on the plans of the physicians and/or new owners (retiring, relocating, becoming employed by the new practice).

Accounts Receivable

Accounts receivable are not typically purchased by new owners (see Chapter 1). Depending on the complexity of the balances (eg, collections, payment plans), pursuing those amounts can usually be accommodated by an outside billing company or on a part-time basis, and possibly from a staff member's home, if you can move the practice's computer there. This arrangement also necessitates that the bank account be open beyond the actual closing date to receive deposits.

An alternative is to sell the accounts receivable to whoever takes over the practice. If this is an option, the selling price of the practice would need to include these balances. This plan is attractive in some situations because it allows the buyers to have cash flow from the first day of operation.

Accounts Payable

All liabilities incurred before the sale's closing date are important. In most instances, the accounts payable remain the obligation of the previous owners and the new owners would not be subject to these claims. As discussed in Chapter 1, a list of all accounts payable by vendor, carryover, or contingent liabilities should be added as an exhibit to the purchase agreement.

Tax Considerations

Sellers of the practice must consider many tax implications. A qualified tax accountant can advise and assist with these matters, including property, payroll, and income taxes, so that appropriate steps may be taken well in advance of the practice dissolution. A more thorough discussion is included in Chapter 1.

Legal Entity Termination

As discussed in previous chapters, the sale of the practice does not automatically dissolve the previous legal entity. The corporation, partnership, or limited liability company must be officially dissolved with the help of legal counsel to ensure compliance with local, state, and federal requirements.

In a group practice, it is likely that physicians would have an employment or shareholder's agreement that spells out the terms of retirement. This agreement would outline salary and ownership interest, place a value on the intangible aspects of the practice, and define the value of the practice's hard assets to which retiring physicians are entitled. Although placing a value on the tangible assets may be relatively simple, much of the practice's value is intangible, based on goodwill that the physician has developed over many years of practicing in the community. Dissolution of the business partnership also has specific requirements for consideration:

- Confirm that the partnership is completely and correctly dissolved, otherwise any obligations under the original agreement will continue.
- Ensure that all parties have performed their duties under the original agreement before signing the dissolution. Once the dissolution has been signed, the original agreement is void.
- File the dissolution statement with the government agency with which the business was originally registered.
- Terminate or transfer all permits, licenses, and fictitious business name registrations.
- Provide written notice of the dissolution to all vendors to notify them that the partners are no longer responsible for each other's debts and obligations. This should be done by the partner initiation dissolution.
- Examine leases, loan agreements, and other contracts to determine how the dissolution will affect them, as some agreements are voided if the partnership dissolves.
- Complete payroll tax deposits and employment tax paperwork on time. Inform all local, state, and federal tax agencies about the dissolution of the business.
- Understand the serious tax implications of dissolution.
- Give all parties time to review the dissolution documents and to have counsel review it as well. Each party should receive a signed, original copy of the dissolution.

Dissolution can become more complicated if the buying physicians are purchasing the practice over time rather than paying for it all at once. It is generally unlawful for one practitioner to pay another practitioner for referrals, as most states have fee-splitting statutes that prevent this. It is possible to structure an arrangement to stay within safe legal boundaries when retiring physicians are involved.

Obviously, some components of the practice may carry over beyond the sale date, such as outstanding liabilities and accounts receivable. The legal entity may continue in transition up to one year to resolve these outstanding matters. Again, appropriate legal counsel should be consulted regarding the appropriate actions.

Transitioning to New Owners

Patients

Patients, of course, are the lifeline of the medical practice. The doctor-patient relationship creates a strong bond, especially in a practice that has been in operation for many years. It is important to inform patients as quickly as possible when the sale of the practice is imminent, so that there is plenty of time to transition to new physicians. Formal notice to the patients should be mailed, with clear instructions about the options for continuing care with other physicians and for retrieving medical records.

The letter serves a dual purpose. First, it notifies patients of the departing physicians' exit date, reason for closing, names of physicians willing to accept new patients, where the medical records will be stored and how copies can be obtained or transferred to another physician, and an authorization form to release records from the practice. The letter provides an opportunity for departing physicians to thank their patients for their trust and patronage while in practice. It is also used to introduce new physicians who may be taking over the practice, setting forth their outstanding credentials, and other endorsements. Examples of termination letters are available in Chapter 1 (Figure 1-6) and Chapter 5 (Figure 5-5). These letters do not need to be sent by certified or registered mail. The requirement is to make a reasonable attempt to notify patients, so regular mail is sufficient. However, high-risk patients may be better served by sending them the letter by certified or registered mail with a request for a return receipt.

According to an article from the law firm of Abrams, Fensterman, Fensterman, Eisman, Greenberg, Formato & Einiger, LLP:

> It is important to note that the sale of a physician's medical practice should not include the sale of medical records, which is prohibited in most states. A physician may not sell his/her medical records as part of the transfer of the practice since those records and the information contained therein are confidential. Typically, the purchasing physician becomes the custodian of the patients' medical records. This means that the records will be retained by the purchasing physician for the relevant statutory period depending on individual state laws. After this time, a copy of the records will be made available to the patient if they wish to see another physician. Until the patient authorizes or consents to treatment, the purchasing physician may not review the patient's medical chart. This authorization may be express (written) or implied (when the patient comes in for an appointment).[1]

In the case of solo practitioners, the individual physician owns the original paper record and the patient has a right to access the information contained in the record. However, in the case of a clinic with two or more physicians, the clinic rather than the individual physicians generally retains possession of the original paper records. Therefore, when an individual physician leaves the practice, the records remain with the clinic, and the patient can request copies of the record as needed.

As addressed in Chapter 5, physicians who have electronic health records rather than paper medical records must still comply with the laws regarding medical record retention and patient access. These laws may require that records be retained for several years after the close of the practice.

Managed Care Organizations

A clear understanding of the managed care plans accepted in the area will help new physicians decide which networks they may need to join. In many cases, the contract will be between the individual physician and the plan and is not generally transferable to a new owner. If the new physician is not an approved provider within the seller's managed care network(s), the contract is of no value, and thus, a purchasing physician must discount the managed care patients of the practice when determining the number of transferable patients. However, if the purchasing physician is an approved provider within the same managed care network, the purchasing physician should be able to continue treating these patients, which would make the managed care contract an asset.

Selling physicians should carefully review all managed care contracts to determine if the agreements are assumable or may be terminated by the payer and also to identify the appropriate process for notifying the plan about the close of the practice. In the case of primary care physicians who may have patients assigned to them, most plans require a minimum of 60 days to reassign those patients to other local physicians.

Personnel

Personnel issues likely entail the most work in practice transitions. Because most employees have an emotional investment in the practice, it is important to recognize the impact that closing the practice may have on them, both emotionally and financially. As discussed in Chapter 1, finding the perfect time to announce the closing of the practice is key to a more successful transition. A clearly defined plan to address typical human resource issues should be outlined well in advance of the closing announcement to the staff. Having clearly defined employee policies that address the termination process is advised.

The new practice owners should decide which employees they may wish to retain or rehire for the new organization. Patients are likely to feel more comfortable in the new practice if they "recognize" a staff member. These actions are discussed in the following sections.

Employee Hiring and Firing

Physicians should have a clear policy regarding employment references—whether to give limited references for all employees or a complete reference that would include employee performance information. There are significant liabilities associated with references; complete references should be handled with caution. The specifics of hiring and firing are discussed in detail in Chapter 1.

Record Keeping

Sellers are subject to wage and hour audits for all employees. They must maintain all human resource records and documentation (eg, salaries, overtime, and time off).

Health Insurance Benefits

Depending on the number of employees, the new owner may be subject to a continuation of coverage under the provisions of Consolidated Omnibus Budget Reconciliation Act (COBRA) regulations. More information about these provisions is found in Chapter 1.

Other Benefits

The entire menu of benefits that is offered to employees by the sellers (eg, sick leave, disability insurance, retirement benefits, life insurance) should be considered by the new practice owners. This does not mean that the new owners have to offer the same benefits package, but the current package should be reviewed to determine how it compares to the benefits package planned for the new practice. When physician owners sell to a larger health system (eg, a hospital, private corporation) with a comprehensive benefits plan, the benefits menu may be substantially better than what was offered in the private practice

The Phase-out Agreement

As discussed in Chapter 1, a well-drafted phase-out agreement can both terminate the parties' commitments and help prevent future misunderstandings and disputes. Through this document, a phase-in buyer or phase-out seller is arranging for both parties to work together.

The phase-out agreement should do the following:

- Address whether one or more partners can continue to operate the practice under the original name.
- Address assumption of legal responsibility for the purchase, rent, or lease of the building and medical equipment.
- Define how long the selling physician will remain in the practice and the level of compensation (including fringe benefits).
- Define the duties of the buyer and seller. (Patient distribution and hours worked should be considered. It must be very clear that in case of disagreement, the new owners will prevail.)

- Establish the actual purchase price by conducting an independent valuation.
- Arrange for parties to exchange monies (at least in deposit form or as earnest money placed in escrow) prior to the official closing during the phase-out period.
- Enable the purchaser to assume more responsibility as time passes. (Purchasing physicians should care for more patients, each getting to know the other, while the selling physicians' role and workload is decreasing.)
- Specify the timeline of the sale. For example, some phase-out agreements last up to five years. If during that period the selling physician agrees to work three days a week and the buyer agrees to work five days a week, this arrangement must be stated, with income allocations based on productivity and cost.

Conclusion

A refocus on hospital-physician consolidation and integration strategies has created a heightened awareness for individual physicians in solo and group practices who are considering retiring or selling their practices. As physicians consider the salability of their practice and try to gauge the optimum time to sell, they also confront the emotional side of closing their practice and terminating the relationships that have been built over years, sometimes many years, with their patients. Physicians planning to transfer or close their medical practice due to retirement, relocation, or in anticipation of the changing health care environment must consider multiple factors and prioritize efforts to ensure minimum stress and maximum value for the practice. Physicians also have ethical and legal considerations that cannot be underestimated or minimized.

Careful planning is the key to successfully closing or transferring a practice to new physicians. By looking at all of the elements involved in closing a practice, physicians can create a carefully orchestrated timeline to eliminate missing important steps along the way. The decision to close a practice by retiring, relocating, or selling to another entity is very important and should involve a long-term strategy rather than a short-term decision. Physicians should seek counsel from trusted professionals, such as attorneys, accountants, tax professionals, and consultants to ensure that they receive the appropriate expert guidance. This action is especially crucial in areas in which they may not have the experience or the time to make sound decisions while continuing to care for patients.

Moreover, careful consideration must be given to ensure that the practice is dissolved efficiently and effectively with as little disruption as possible during the process. Because the process of closure involves a co-mingling in multiple areas, including accounts receivable and accounts payable, it entails serious tax and legal implications. Protection of all tangible and intangible assets, as well as maximizing collections, will ensure the greatest value for the property.

By carefully outlining all responsibilities and following this roadmap for dissolution, fewer areas will be open to interpretation and doubt. In fact, addressing dissolution at the onset of the partnership is also an excellent time to start long-term preparation for retirement or sale of the practice.

Endnote

1. Einiger S. Transferring your medical practice—an often overlooked asset. Available at http://www.abramslaw.com/CM/Articles/Transferring-Your-Medical-Practice-An-Often-Overlooked-Asset.asp. Accessed May 18, 2011.

3

PART THREE

Valuing the Medical Practice

Part 3 equips the reader with understanding the worth of the practice when making informed decisions for the future. Physicians who seek to maximize the value of their practice now will be able to enhance their options later. Regardless of the need for assessment, the reader will gain insight into the process, methods, guidelines, and benefits of practice valuation. These chapters also cover managing the appraiser-client relationship, appraisal regulations, preparing the practice for maximum value, and fair market value opinions.

CHAPTER 7 Concepts of Value

OUTLINE

Physicians, as a group, have various reasons for wanting to know the value of their medical practices. Those reasons can be chiefly dependent on current happenings in the industry or the physicians' present career stage.

Recent developments both in and outside of the industry, such as financial uncertainty, issues related to declining reimbursement resulting from the Patient Protection and Affordable Care Act of 2010, and the ever increasing regulations, have stimulated hospitals and health systems to acquire physician practices. Unlike the acquisitions in the 1990s—when practice management companies, hospitals, and other entities primarily used stock and high levels of compensation to lure physicians into selling their practices—today, the focus is more on the true value of the practice and the ability to support it with fair market standards within regulatory guidelines. While hospitals still see acquisitions as a way of protecting market share, it is imperative that these acquisitions make financial sense for them, as well as for the physicians.

Selling a practice is not the only reason to have a valuation performed. Another reason is when a practice wishes to bring on a new partner. It is likely that a new partner will need to make some type of investment to qualify for ownership. Without a valuation, the figure that represents the value of the practice would have no more meaning than an arbitrary number picked at random. However, everyone can be reasonably sure that the numbers are legitimate when they are derived from a fair and equitable valuation by a qualified, independent third party.

Finally, a valuation may be completed for no other reason than to assess the performance of a practice (ie, as management tools). How would an owner or group of owners measure the achievements or failures of their practice if they have nothing with which to compare it? Of course, numerous benchmarks can provide an excellent road map, but unless a detailed valuation is completed, it cannot be definitively determined where the practice stands. Furthermore, because of the due diligence that must be thoroughly completed to calculate a value, certain operational issues may come to light that would have otherwise gone unnoticed. Thus, valuations can serve as excellent management tools.

Understanding the theory behind the valuation process (as discussed in depth in Chapter 2) requires a good working knowledge of the various revenue rulings, as determined by the Internal Revenue Service (IRS). The IRS revenue rulings serve as the foundation for deriving a valuation of an entity. These revenue rulings—specifically Revenue Ruling 59-60—provide the foundation for virtually all that is discussed in this book and in other books of this nature. Therefore, to understand the processes and methodologies of assessing the value of a medical practice, one must become familiar with the framework used to create those processes and methodologies.

Internal Revenue Service Revenue Ruling 59-60

Revenue Ruling 59-60 (RR 59-60) often has been heralded as the most preeminent document regarding the valuation of a closely held entity. Whether intentional or unintentional, this document was years ahead of its time. RR 59-60 was originally drafted to provide guidance for estate and gift tax valuation purposes. However, throughout the years, it has become the predominant document used to determine valuation processes for all closely held entities.

In a period in which both processes and methodologies are constantly being modified to keep pace with the changes in the business and regulatory environments, this time-tested document from the 1950s has remained constant in the realm of valuations and the valuation process. It has endured as the standard for more than half a century.

RR 59-60 establishes a number of basic concepts and criteria that are still followed today throughout the valuation process. These factors establish the fundamental theory of business valuation, and each deserves diligent analysis and direct application in valuing an entity. The following brief list includes some key components set by RR 59-60[1] that must be considered:

- The nature of the business
- The history of the business from its start
- The economic outlook of the business
- The general condition and outlook of the industry
- The current financial condition of the business
- The earning capacity of the business
- The dividend paying capacity of the company
- The existence of goodwill or other intangible value
- The value of stock for sale or value of blocks of stock within the business
- Market prices of comparable business within the industry, whether stocks are actively traded in a free and open market or sold directly from business to business

While some of these factors are not applicable to the valuation of a medical practice, the appraiser must use a similar approach when valuing any business. It is unimportant whether a practice is a sole proprietorship, a corporation, or a partnership; the value of the business relates to the business conducted and the historical and prospective financial performance of the entity.

Other Revenue Rulings

In addition to RR 59-60, a number of other rulings have greatly affected the manner in which closely held organizations are valued. While some of these may not directly affect the valuation methodologies of a closely held company, such as a solo medical practice, the preponderance of them contribute to the basic theory and assumptions that are used in the valuation process in general.

Some of the more important rulings that affect the valuation of a closely held company and their general contribution to the valuation process include the following:

- *Revenue Ruling 68-609 (RR 68-609).* This ruling describes what is often referred to as the *formula method*; it discusses the utilization of the formula approach in determining the fair market value of the intangible assets of a business only if there is no other suitable method for determining this value. The formula approach is also referred to as the *excess earnings method* (discussed in more depth in Chapter 9). Furthermore, the approach details the method in which the formula method should be based and considerations that should be made in using it, as well as providing language that supersedes Revenue Ruling 65-192 (RR 65-192).[2]

- *Revenue Ruling 77-287 (RR 77-287).* As noted in RR 77-287, "The purpose of this ruling is to amplify Rev. Rul. 59-60 . . . and to provide information and guidance to taxpayers, Internal Revenue Service personnel, and others concerned with the valuation, for Federal tax purposes, of securities that cannot immediately be resold because they are restricted from resale pursuant to Federal securities laws."[3]
- *Revenue Ruling 83-120 (RR 83-120).* This ruling expounds on the valuation process and the factors that must be considered when valuing common and preferred stock. It goes into greater depth in comparison to RR 59-60 in the valuation of preferred stock and the unique considerations that it gains.
- *Revenue Ruling 93-1 (RR 93-1).* This ruling specifically revokes Revenue Ruling 81-253 (RR 81-253) and addresses the issues of transferring ownership shares within a family and corporate control.

While none of these rulings specifically addresses the valuation of a closely held entity, per se, each forms a part of the whole that plays a substantial role in the valuation processes and methodologies.

Approaches to Value

Based on the aforementioned revenue rulings, the three major approaches to valuing a closely held company have been determined to be the market approach, asset-based approach, and the income approach. While these approaches are based on contrastingly different methodologies, in theory, if performed correctly, they should conclude with the same valuation total. This presumption, however, is theoretical; in actuality, the three different methodologies often draw varying conclusions.

Although Chapter 4 details each of the methodologies, brief descriptions of the three approaches are provided in the following sections.

Market Approach

The market approach is based on the theory of substitution and the underlying "premise that a prudent buyer will pay no more for a property than it would cost to acquire a substitute property with the same utility."[4] This methodology applies to a comparative analysis of prices paid for similar assets or an entity in the marketplace. In this approach, the appraiser estimates the value of the entity by applying data from similar companies, called guideline companies, to the same data from the subject company (ie, the company being valued).

This market method must be completed in most cases; unfortunately, it has little applicability to smaller practices (in large part due to the lack of data on these companies and their transactions). However, with the onset of regularly occurring practice purchases and transitions, information that can be applied will undoubtedly improve with time. Currently, for valuation purposes of larger entities, the market approach is an integral portion of the valuation process.

Asset-based Approach

The asset-based approach is often referred to as the cost approach, the adjusted net asset approach, or the adjusted balance sheet approach. For the purposes of this analysis, the term asset-based approach will be used. This method, like that of the market approach, is based on the theory of substitution. However, while the market approach looks outward (ie, to other similar companies) for information to apply inward, the asset-based approach works in the opposite direction. It analyzes an entity's balance sheet and involves the individual valuation of each tangible and intangible asset residing on that entity's balance sheet.

In this approach, intangible assets—or a practice's goodwill—are valued using the excess earnings method. The downfall of this methodology is that if the business has more intangible value, it becomes more difficult to use this approach. Because of the increased intangible value (eg, RR 68-609), this methodology is often included as a supporting value and rarely is used as the final value of an entity, especially in the case of a medical practice or other heavily service-oriented business.

Income Approach

The income approach is considered the closest to pure theory. The fair market value of a company (discussed in Chapter 2) is determined by converting anticipated benefits into current or present value as a return on investment and value of all future benefits of the company. This methodology is the most widely used and accepted approach in valuing a closely held entity. Furthermore, it is best structured to determine the value of a medical practice.

However, as widely used and accepted as the income approach is, it is not faultless. In fact a major downfall to this methodology is that it is highly subjective in the underlying calculations used to reach a conclusive total, thus leaving room for mistakes and errors. If a highly skilled, competent appraiser is completing the process and is familiar with the method, this factor should have little importance once a final value has been reached.

Tangible and Intangible Assets

An entity has two types of assets: tangible and intangible. Each type is discussed in the following sections.

Tangible Assets

An entity's tangible assets are generally the easiest to value because of their physical nature (ie, they can be touched, felt, seen, and easily counted). These assets include equipment, furniture, supplies, and fixtures. Because they are material, the appraiser can more easily associate a price to them. However, tangible assets also include those items that are not so easy to touch or see. These include items such as accounts receivable, cash, contracts, or notes receivable. While these items cannot be seen or held in a manner similar to a desk or an examination table, they are every bit as tangible and valuable.

These items are often confused and difficult to understand; therefore, following are definitions of the common tangible assets within a medical practice.

- Equipment: All capital assets used to assist in the delivery of services within the physician practice are considered equipment. Such items include—but are certainly not limited to—laboratory equipment, diagnostic equipment, examining room equipment, procedure room equipment, and the like.
- Office supplies: While treated as an expense when purchased, most supplies are tangible assets when accumulated. Customarily, a physician's practice keeps a minimum of a one-month stock of office and medical supplies.
- Office furniture: Tangible furniture includes desks, chairs, filing cabinets, etc.
- Accounts receivable: Accounts receivable are those monies due from patients, insurance companies, and other creditors as a result of services provided within the practice.
- Contracts of long-term (notes) receivables: These assets include contracts from long-term, income-generating projects within the practice.

- Leasehold improvements: These assets are items added to the existing leased structure that may include plumbing, electrical, or other items of improvement. Typically, these items are permanently attached to the structure and are not removable when the lease ends.
- Office building and land: The cost of the building and the land associated with the practice are tangible. Often, these are owned by separate entities and are leased back to the practice. Furthermore, if they are not directly part of the practice and its operations, these will warrant a separate real estate appraisal.
- Cash and cash equivalents: This asset includes any cash on-hand within the practice's bank accounts, money market accounts, or any other extremely liquid vehicles. Cash equivalents are those items such as securities or other semi-liquid vehicles.
- Automobiles: When owned by the practice, automobiles represent tangible value and should be treated as such, if they are to be included in the sale of the practice.
- Investments: These assets include valid insurance policies and the market value of investments.
- Leases: These assets may include any current capital leases entered into by the practice.

Intangible Assets

While tangible assets are those that can be seen, touched, and easily identified, intangible assets are just the opposite. They cannot be seen or touched and are often difficult to identify and value. Also, they are the most misunderstood aspects of the valuation of an entity. Intangible assets fall into two broad categories: *apart from goodwill* and *goodwill.*

Apart From Goodwill

Intangible value apart from goodwill includes those assets that can be separated from the practice. They may include patient credit records, leasehold interests, trademarks, copyrights, patents, franchises, restrictive covenants, and the value of managed care contracting rights. Intangible assets can be separated from the practice because they have a definable cost basis and reasonable life expectancy separate from goodwill. If relevant, the appraiser considers the intangible value of these assets.

Goodwill

Goodwill is generally referred to as an intangible asset that cannot be separated from the practice. Unfortunately, this term causes confusion and remains difficult to explain. Even within the realms of experienced appraisers, this term evokes distinct variances of opinion and even controversies. However, the calculation of goodwill is most often the inherent value that we are trying to determine.

In larger organizations, such as those actively traded on public stock exchanges, goodwill is often referred to as the difference between the market value of the organization (ie, the total number of shares outstanding multiplied by the current price per share) less the tangible assets of the organization. Clearly, in a privately held entity, this valuation would be difficult to determine due to the lack of a readily available price per share.

In some cases, companies would "amortize goodwill, writing it off in relatively small, regular chunks each quarter over a period of years or decades until it was gone."[4] This practice commonly occurs in larger organizations such as hospitals and not in smaller physician practices. However, Statements 141 and 142 from the Financial Accounting Standards Board (FASB) indicate that the method in which this goodwill is being carried on an entity's balance sheet is changed. Accordingly, companies "can now keep goodwill on their balance sheets indefinitely. But they must perform annual tests to see if the goodwill has become 'impaired,' that is, if it has suffered a permanent decline in value. If it has, they must write off the entire impaired amount resulting in sometimes large"[5] changes in the amounts of goodwill the company can claim on its balance sheet. This goodwill and the treatment thereof is something that the appraiser must certainly consider.

Because it is the goal of the appraiser to value the goodwill of the entity, the appraiser must fully understand the concept of goodwill and how it applies to a company.

Conclusion

This chapter lays the groundwork for the in-depth review of the processes and methodologies that follow. Appraisers must understand the theory and the basis for which the valuation is completed, and they must be knowledgeable of the foundation on which these processes and methodologies have been constructed.

The completion of a valuation is much more than the entering of numbers into a formula to determine the value of an entity. While a valuation's roots are based in accounting, largely on accounting fundamentals, completing a valuation is less clear cut and more related to theories and assumptions. Thus, appraisers will often find that general certified public accountants (CPAs) with little or no experience in the valuation field have an extraordinarily difficult time in understanding the abstract thought that must be applied to the valuation process.

However, this is not to discount the necessity for being able to understand and competently navigate a corporation's financial statements, for without this, there will be no foundation on which to base the valuation theories.

Therefore, it is not the purpose of this book to teach the most basic financial operations, because a thorough working knowledge of these issues must already be known. The intent of this book is to offer the additional knowledge and expertise needed to lay the groundwork for someone educated in these areas to perform a quality appraisal of a business entity.

Endnotes

1. Internal Revenue Service. Revenue Ruling 59–60. Available at http://www.hantzmonwiebel.com/live_data/documents/ruling-59-60.pdf. Accessed June 10, 2011.
2. Formula Method of Valuation, Revenue Ruling 68-609. http://www.equityvaluations.com/pubs/revenueruling68-609.html. Accessed June 9, 2011.
3. Internal Revenue Service. Revenue Ruling 77–287. Available at http://www.businessvalue.com/resources/Valuation-Cases/Revenue-Ruling-77-287.pdf. Accessed June 10, 2011.
4. American Society of Appraisers. Introduction to Business Valuation, Part 1. In: *Principles of Valuation: Business Valuation Student Manual, BV 201.* Herndon, VA: American Society of Appraisers; 2002:7.
5. Casey EW, Wist B, et al. KPMG White Paper. *Accounting for Business Combinations, Goodwill, and Intangible Assets: An Analysis of FASB Statements 141 and 142.* New York, NY: KPMG LLP; 2001.

CHAPTER 8 Valuation Process

OUTLINE

I. Introduction
II. Define the Appraisal Assignment
  A. Basis of Value
  B. Standard of Value
    1. Fair Market Valuation
    2. Fair Value
    3. Investment Value
    4. Intrinsic Value
  C. Purpose for Valuation
III. Type of Appraisal
  A. Appraisal
  B. Limited Appraisal
  C. Calculations
  D. Hypothetical Appraisal
IV. Letter of Engagement
  A. Other Agreements
  B. Appraisal Fee
V. Conclusion

Understanding the theory behind the valuation process allows one to understand the manner in which the valuation process should be completed. Completing the valuation process thoroughly and following the steps integral to this process will ensure that all relevant issues are addressed and resolved properly.

The American Society of Appraisers (ASA) has outlined the following five steps of the valuation process[1]:

1. Define the appraisal assignment
2. Gather the data

3. Analyze the data
4. Arrive at the valuation conclusion (ie, a value)
5. Write the report

Every valuation is unique and, while similarities exist, it is not likely that any one valuation will be exactly the same. Generally, but not in all situations, the five steps will apply. The focus of this chapter is on the first step: define the appraisal assignment and draft the agreement.

Define the Appraisal Assignment

The valuation process begins by defining the appraisal assignment, which is then incorporated into the letter of agreement stating and outlining the work that will be done. In developing a business valuation, an appraiser must identify and define the following valuation components:

- The basis of value (ie, business, business ownership interest, or security to be valued)
- The effective date of the appraisal (ie, the "as of" date)
- The standard of value (ie, what kind of value is desired)
- The purpose and the intended use of the valuation (somewhat similar to the standard of value)

The nature and scope of the assignment must be defined. Acceptable scopes of work will generally be one of three types: appraisal, limited appraisal, or calculations.

Basis of Value

To determine the basis of value, the appraiser must ask, "What is going to be valued?" This question may seem elementary—for who would ask for a valuation when they do not even know what they want valued—but it is more complex. Understanding what entity is going to be valued is fairly straightforward. If a physician wants the practice valued, then the appraiser will know to value the practice and everything that falls under the spectrum of the practice. The difficult part for the appraiser will be determining what portion of that entity will be valued.

In the case of a solo practitioner's practice, the practitioner may wish to only sell a portion of the practice. What if that portion equals a 75% interest? What if that portion equals only a 33% interest? When valuing a single physician's interest in a large, multispecialty practice owned by a number of physicians, the appraiser must know implicitly what portion of this interest is being valued and what this encompasses. The value of the whole may significantly differ from the value of a fraction, regardless of whether it is a large multispecialty practice or a solo practitioner's practice.

As the ASA notes, "The different valuation approaches and methods used in a business appraisal produce different indications of value by the very nature of the empirical data used in the approach or method."[2]

The three bases of values that the appraiser must consider are *minority marketable*, *control*, and *minority nonmarketable* bases of value. The type of valuation that is completed will depend on the basis that is considered.

When considered in the terms of completing a valuation, the ideas of control and minority value are relatively easy to understand, and the theory behind the basis of value is quite logical. First, consider the difference between a control and a minority valuation. A *control valuation* is a valuation of a company, or portion thereof, which can be readily and easily affected by the owner of what is being valued. This will almost always be a private, or closely held company, because the ownership of this entity will have considerable control over the plight of that company.

Think of the case, for example, in which a large family practice clinic is being appraised. This practice started with one physician, and that physician has retained 100% of the ownership. That one physician has considerable control over the direction and management of the practice. If an individual were to purchase the practice (ie, 100% of the practice), then this would be considered a control valuation. Thus, it is likely that the purchaser would pay a premium for the ability to have direct control over the business. Conversely, this ownership interest would have very little liquidity (ie, marketability) associated with it. This is because it does not trade freely on an open stock exchange or some other market and it cannot be easily divested, as opposed to a share of a publicly traded stock, which can be quickly and efficiently bought and sold many times over. This lack of liquidity may call for a corresponding discount or decrease in value.

Now consider the opposite situation, in which a physician's practice was purchased by a publicly traded physician practice management company (PPMC) and, in this purchase, the physician was granted an ownership portion of the PPMC. A number of other practices were bought as well, and these physicians were also made shareholders, totaling 1,000 physician owners of the PPMC. If one physician chooses to sell his or her portion, this would be considered a minority basis of valuation, because that one physician has very little control over the day-to-day decision-making process and his or her actions could not significantly affect the plight of the company.

In this situation, an analyst would likely assert a discount to this minority stake. Although, as in the case of the control valuation, in which the ownership interest being valued was assumed to be relatively illiquid, and which will most generally be the case, the minority share can be either highly liquid or highly illiquid. In the aforementioned example, the ownership portion would likely be very liquid, or marketable, meaning that it could easily and readily be transferred to another owner, like the ownership of stock in a public company. This is referred to as a minority marketable basis of value.

Now consider a similar example. Instead of a large group of physicians, this group consists of four providers, and a minority share of one provider must be appraised. In this case, it may be more difficult to exchange or relinquish that individual's ownership share, thus rendering it less marketable. This would be considered a minority nonmarketable basis of valuation. A discount for both minority ownership and lack of marketability may be considered.

As pointed out in the examples in this section, it is evident that an appraiser must be aware of the entity that is being valued to properly conduct the valuation.

Standard of Value

The next step in the valuation process is determining what kind of value is desired. The answer will largely be determined by the answer to another question: What is the purpose of this valuation? The answers to these two key questions must be addressed before progress can be made.

As noted in Chapter 1, valuations are not completed only when someone wants to buy or sell an entity or a portion of an entity. There are numerous reasons as to why an entity may require a valuation, including the transfer of ownership (ie, buying or selling) of a company. A few of the more common reasons for conducting a valuation include the following:

- Buying or selling
- Tax related
- Financial reporting
- Legal issues
- Divorce
- Damages, etc
- Internal issues
- Buy/sell agreements
- Stock distributions
- Adding/disengaging a partner

While there are numerous reasons why an appraisal must be performed, the end use of the appraisal must be clear to determine the appropriate standard of valuation.

Fair Market Valuation

Fair market valuation is defined in Revenue Ruling 59-60 (RR 59-60) from the Internal Revenue Service (IRS) as "the amount at which the property would change hands between a willing buyer and a willing seller, when the former is not under any compulsion to buy and the latter is not under any compulsion to sell; both parties having reasonable knowledge of relevant facts."[3] The five characteristics of a market value are as follows[4]:

1. The buyer and seller are typically motivated.
2. Both parties are well informed or well advised and acting in what they consider their best interests.
3. A reasonable time is allowed for exposure in the open market.
4. Payment is made in terms of cash or financial arrangements comparable thereto.
5. The price represents the normal consideration for the property sold unaffected by special or creative financing or sales concessions granted by anyone associated with the sale.

Although the terms *market value* and *cash value* are used interchangeably, *fair market value* is not to be confused with *fair value*.

Fair market value will be addressed extensively in Chapter 14.

Fair Value

The term *fair value* can be used in two different instances: legal and financial. For legal purposes, fair value is usually that which is determined by a court of law; it does not have to be associated with fair market value. Fair value and the calculation that results usually vary based on state laws and regulations and bear little resemblance to fair market value. Furthermore, due to its various meanings, there is little uniformity in the definition of fair legal value. In cases of fair legal value, there does not have to be a willing buyer or seller. These valuations are most often used in cases of shareholder dissent or minority oppression cases. With regard to financial reporting, fair value is more strongly associated with tax and generally accepted accounting principles than with valuation terms.

Investment Value

Investment value is the specific value of goods or services to a particular investor (or class of investors) based on individual investment requirements and expectation. The investment value often calculates a different value than the fair market value. In determining fair market value, the buyer and seller are equals; however, when calculating the investment value of an entity, one side of the equation (ie, the buyer or the seller) may have significantly different reasons for wanting to make such an investment. No specific reason exists for why an entity may be of more value to one particular owner than to another; in fact, there may be myriad reasons.

The basic premise behind the determination of investment value is the assumptions used to determine this value. When determining investment value over fair market value, the assumptions will generally be skewed to meet the predetermined standards set by the investor.

Intrinsic Value

Intrinsic value is often referred to as *fundamental value.* This "represents an analytical judgment of value based on the perceived characteristics inherent in the investment, not tempered by characteristics peculiar to one investor, but rather tempered by how these perceived characteristics are interpreted by one analyst versus another."[5] In essence, intrinsic value is fair market value with the variances caused by the market (ie, supply and demand) removed.

Intrinsic value is often used in stock analysis of a company. For instance, the statement may be that "The stock price has been lowered, but its fundamentals still look good." This means that the supply or demand for the stock has caused it to lose value, but the actual value of the stock remains sound. So for a publicly traded stock in the market, a stock analyst would likely consider this devalued stock a "buy."

Purpose for Valuation

The next step in the valuation process is determining the purpose for the valuation. The purpose for valuation and the standard of value are similar to the "chicken and egg" conundrum (ie, which one came first; to know one, the other must also be known). The various purposes for valuating an entity lead to different ways to determine the standard of value that will be used.

An entity may consider completing a valuation for numerous reasons. The most obvious reason for performing a valuation is to determine the value of an entity for the purpose of buying or selling it. Another reason may be for tax purposes, so that tax implications (eg, IRS assessed excise or estate taxes) can be determined.

Yet another reason for completing a valuation is for legal purposes. When determining the value for legal reasons, the court will often specify a fair value, not fair market value. Legal purposes are most often used in divorce or dissenting shareholder cases, although value may be determined for other reasons. Legal purposes can also be used to assess damages to one party or for partnership dissolutions. While the reasons can be varying, these valuations can often be burdened by legal and other complexities, making some appraisers somewhat reluctant to assume these types of projects.

Probably the most common reason for determining the value of an entity or a portion thereof is for internal reasons (eg, for financial reporting, buy/sell agreements, stock distributions, adding/leaving partner). Determining the valuation for internal purposes is particularly important for closely held companies. In this case, the shareholders do not have the luxury of finding out their current stock value just by looking on the Internet, as would the owner of a publicly held company. Instead, these physicians must determine the value of their company based on an appraisal.

Also, buy/sell agreements will often call for an updated valuation to be completed when a new shareholder is added. While these agreements will often be limited as to when they can be executed to correspond with the prearranged valuation, if they are not, it is certainly in the interest of both the current shareholders and the new shareholder to know the value of the stock at the time of purchase.

Closely held companies will often include a valuation of their company with the annual financial statements. The price of a company's stock is a great barometer for determining the performance of the company. Without the benefit of easily being able to find this out (ie, through public information), a valuation often serves as an excellent supplement to a company's annual financial documents.

One can see how an appraiser must know what they are valuing to establish the standard of value that will be used. If an appraiser has been contracted by an individual who seeks to purchase a medical practice in a particular city or area of the country, that individual may be willing to pay a little more than a practice's fair market value to get what they want. For this reason, the appropriate standard for valuation in this case would likely be the investment value. However, if a board of directors wanted to see how their company's value had increased since the last year, they may be more interested in the intrinsic value than the fair market value.

Before the valuation process can begin, the appraiser *must* know why this valuation is being completed. This answer will serve as the foundation for all of the assumptions made in calculating the value.

Type of Appraisal

This section describes what is necessary to complete an appraisal of a medical entity. It should be noted, however, that a full appraisal is not always what is needed or required by the client.

Often, a potential client will contact an appraiser and ask for a valuation of a specific entity but not a full valuation. For example, when a physician wishes to buy into a practice and the physician owners offer a buy-in price, the prospective partner will want to validate that number. In this case, the prospective partner may choose to hire an appraiser to determine if the asking price is valid and falls within the realm of reasonableness. The prospective partner may ask for a limited appraisal just to "run the numbers" and determine if the offer is within reason.

Another example of why an appraisal might be conducted is when an entity wants to know the company's value based on the prospect of certain events or changes in the company. This would be considered a *pro forma* or *hypothetical valuation*.

While these initiatives vary significantly from a full valuation, there is nothing that makes completing these appraisals unethical to the appraiser. However, the appraiser must make it known that this is what the client has asked to be done, and that this is all that will be completed. This type of appraisal must be stated clearly and be understood by both parties before an agreement to complete a valuation is executed.

Appraisal

"The objective of an appraisal is to express an unambiguous opinion about the value of the business...which is supported by all procedures that the appraiser deems to be relevant to the valuation."[6] An appraisal is a valuation that considers all aspects of the business and considers—but does not necessarily apply—all methods of valuation (ie, income, market, asset-based) to determine the value of an entity.

An appraisal will clearly state the conclusions of the appraisal analysis (ie, the value of the entity) based on all relevant information as of the appraisal date. The conclusion, or value, can be stated based on a defined, exact figure, or it can be expressed as a range. Which way the value is expressed must be clearly agreed upon between the appraiser and the client. In addition to the conclusion itself, the information used to calculate the appraisal conclusion will be outlined in detail. The procedures and methodology used to collect, analyze, and reach the conclusion will also be outlined. Finally, an appraisal will *consider* all of the approaches to valuation.

Notice the emphasis on consider in the previous sentence. Although all of the approaches to value must be *considered*, this does not mean that the appraiser must apply all of the approaches. It is the discretion of the appraiser to apply the most appropriate approach.

For example, a physician's office will likely have very few assets (ie, tangible, intangible), so it *may* not be appropriate to apply the asset-based approach to value. Whether an approach is to be applied, as has been stated, is the sole discretion of the appraiser. Of course, the choice to include or exclude a particular approach to value must be an educated decision, not just the analyst's decision to disregard one particular approach. If the analyst chooses not to apply one approach, the reasoning for doing so must be fully defendable.

Limited Appraisal

The limited appraisal is very similar to an appraisal; however, due to their differences, the appraiser is required to note that the calculations that have been used are limited in nature. This is usually (although not always) necessary due to the fact that the appraiser has not been given access to all the data needed to complete an appraisal.

A limited appraisal will fully document the value of the entity (as either an exact amount or a range), with the appraiser considering all three approaches to value. The differences between the limited appraisal and the appraisal are in the information gathering, research, and analysis of the valuation process (often referred to as *due diligence*), in that the appraiser has based the valuation conclusions on limited relevant information, or completed only a limited due diligence process. Regardless of why or which process has been limited in nature, all processes needed to complete an appraisal have not been met. The outcome, therefore, will be a limited appraisal.

Because an appraisal is limited in nature does not mean that it is not "right." In fact, the client may desire to have a limited appraisal completed. If so, this arrangement should be clearly defined in the letter of engagement and agreed upon by the appraiser and the client. In addition, the fact that this appraisal is limited in nature should be clearly stated in the report. The worse thing that could happen between an appraiser and a client is for the client to think that an appraisal has been completed, when in fact only a limited appraisal has been done. In such a case, both individuals will likely walk away from the appraisal with embarrassment.

Calculations

A *calculation* expresses the value of an entity (either as one figure or a range of figures). It is similar to the limited appraisal in that it can be based on limited data and a limited data-collection process. It differs, however, in its approach to value. In the case of the calculation, the appraiser and the client will usually agree upon the type of approach to value that will be used prior to the appraisal.

Typically, an analysis on this level will be for the client and used for informational purposes. For example, clients may request that an appraiser value their entity based only on a financial analysis (ie, no review of operations, thus limiting the due diligence that has been dedicated to this assignment) and using the income approach. This approach could be chosen because it was used five years ago when the practice was valued and the owners want to see, based strictly on a financial review, if the value of the practice has appreciated or declined.

Again, a valuation for this purpose can be completed, although it must be expressly agreed upon by the client and defined by the appraiser within the report.

Hypothetical Appraisal

Appraisals, limited appraisals, and calculations are based on reasonable assumptions that best resemble the future operations of the entity being valued. However, the client may choose to see not the value of the entity under the most reasonable assumptions for future operations but under assumptions as to potential future operations, or pro forma.

A client may wish to see what the value of the practice will be if staff increases productivity by 50% rather than the likely growth rate of 10%. Alternatively, the client may choose to see the value if the provider compensation decreased rather than increased by 5% per year. These are examples of hypothetical scenarios (ie, scenarios that do not coincide with projected future operations as determined by the appraiser) that are used to calculate the value of an entity.

Often, a client will request that an appraiser complete an appraisal of the entity and, in addition to the appraisal, determine what will happen to the value if other scenarios are applied. A hypothetical appraisal can be an appraisal, a limited appraisal, or just based on calculations. These types of appraisals are often useful planning tools for the client, although regardless of their intended use, it must be fully documented that they are hypothetical. If an appraiser is acting as an independent analyst and basing the calculations on his or her own independently formulated assumptions, it is very important to note that the appraisal is hypothetical, due to the fact that most hypothetical appraisals are based on assumptions dictated by the client or a representative of the client. Thus, failure to note that the appraisal is hypothetical could drastically impugn the independence of the appraiser.

Letter of Engagement

Before any valuation work can be completed, the client requiring the valuation must request the services of a valuation professional. This request is typically memorialized in a *request for services letter* or *letter of engagement* between the professional (ie, usually the firm that employs the appraiser) and the client.

This letter of engagement should be thorough in its scope, expressly defining all of the details of the potential project. This letter is very important because it lays the foundation for the future project.

In general, and certainly depending on the size and scope of the valuation that will be completed, the letter of engagement will go through a number of changes and modifications to properly define all that is necessary to complete the project. Reasons for this may vary, but these changes and modifications take place so that the project can be properly defined, as based on the desires of the client.

On larger projects, the drafting of the letter of engagement will typically be the result of numerous meetings—both on-site and off-site—between the client and the appraiser. These meetings will allow the professional to better define that which the client desires to be completed. Thus, because the appraiser and the client have been able to discuss the many aspects of minutiae contained (and required) in the letter of engagement, it is less likely that the letter of engagement will require as many, if any, modifications.

In the case of a smaller-sized medical practice, the letter of engagement may be the result of only a single telephone call or brief meeting. In such cases the appraiser may have limited information about what the client needs, or simply may have misinterpreted what the client needs, thus, changes and modifications may be required. There is nothing wrong or unethical about making changes or modifications to the letter of engagement; however, *after* the agreement has been consummated, making changes to the letter of engagement is highly unprofessional and should never occur. Revisions before signing the agreement are virtually always required because once the letter of engagement has been executed by all of the necessary parties, it shall stand as a legally binding and enforceable contract. Any breach should be regarded as a breach of contract.

It is understandable that issues will arise that will potentially change that which has been defined in the letter of engagement. In such cases it may be necessary to supplement or update the original letter of engagement, again, expressly outlining the details involved, the reason for the changes, and agreement by all parties involved.

Figure 8-1 is an example of a letter of engagement for a medium-sized medical practice. This figure contains all of the necessary information that must be agreed upon by the client and the appraiser, such as the basis of value, the standard of value that will be applied, the type of appraisal, the purpose of the appraisal, who will be completing the appraisal, when it will be completed, the type of value that will be provided (ie, an exact figure or a range), the fees that will be charged to the client, and more.

As previously noted, to complete a full appraisal, the analyst must fully understand the operations of the entity that will be valued; thus, the analyst must complete a review of not only the entity's financials, but also its basic operations (eg, management, daily operations, long-term planning). Because this review must be completed, the client has an excellent opportunity to furnish both a detailed valuation and an assessment of the entity's operations. This review is often more involved than a typical appraisal and will take more of the analyst's time, thereby increasing the cost to the client. In addition, the professional completing the valuation must not only be knowledgeable in the field of valuations but also in the area of business that is in question, specifically medical practice management and operations.

Someone not intimate with the operations of a medical practice or a hospital, for example, would certainly be able to complete the financial

Letter of Engagement

Healthcare Appraisers, LLC (the "Appraiser"), is pleased to present Atlanta Orthopedic Physicians, PA (the "Client"), the practice of John D. Smith, MD, and Bob A. Jones, MD (the "Physicians"), with this Letter of Engagement ("Letter") to outline the Appraiser's proposed approach to the completion of the Valuation and Assessment ("Valuation") of South Atlanta Orthopedics and Physical Therapy, LLC (the "Practice"). This Letter shall consist of Appraiser's:

- Understanding of the issues
- Proposed method of completion
- Summary of fees

Understanding of the Issues

Appraiser understands that the Client wishes to purchase the controlling (100%) ownership interest of the Practice in the South Atlanta area. The Client is requesting that Appraiser complete a valuation and assessment, as defined below, of the Practice in order to determine a price that may be offered to the Practice by the Client.

Proposed Method of Completion

Appraiser has divided the proposed method of completion into two categories: Project I and Project II. Both of these Projects comprise the detailed Valuation of the Practice. They are defined as follows: Project I: Practice Valuation and Limited Assessment Project I shall consist of a detailed valuation and limited operational assessment of the Practice. This review shall encompass the ongoing operations and associated revenue generated by the Practice. This includes a review of its current operations, with special emphasis on its historical performance trends and overall estimates of future performance. This review will include a limited operational assessment that will allow Appraiser to gain a better perspective of the Practice's financial operations.

The intent of this review is to determine the fair market value of the Practice via a full appraisal. The independently derived value will serve as the standard for determining the potential sale/acquisition price of the Practice and will be proposed as a single dollar figure. The completion of this process is independent—that is, without influence from either side (ie, the Client and the Practice)—however, it shall be completed on behalf of the Client.

Phase One

Initial Assessment and Review of Information Off Site. Appraiser will commence its review of the Practice by submitting a checklist of information. Upon submission, Appraiser will review this in preparation of on-site work.

Professional Fees

Estimated hours to complete this phase:

x to x hours @ $xxx per hour $xxx to $xxx

FIGURE 8-1 Letter of Engagement

Source: *Assessing the Value of the Medical Practice,* 2nd ed.

Phase Two

On-site Review. Appraiser will conduct an on-site review of the Practice encompassing analysis of operations in the context of the definition of this assignment review. Appraiser will complete this work by meeting with the physician/owner and other appropriate representatives of the practice and reviewing all key areas inherent to the scope of this assignment. From the work completed during this on-site review, Appraiser will then be prepared to complete the actual independent Valuation report within the context of this assignment.

Professional Fees

Estimated hours to complete this phase:

x to x days on-site @ $xxx per day* (one consultant) $xxx to $xxx

Phase Three

Formal Report. After completing Phases One and Two, Appraiser will be prepared to complete the formal report, indicating the valuation conclusions. Furthermore, this report will include a limited operational assessment of the Practice as noted above. This phase will include the compilation and submission of that formal report documenting this information.

Professional Fees

Estimated hours to complete this phase:

x to x hours @ $xxx per hour $xxx to $xxx

Project II: Detailed Operational Assessment

Project II shall consist of a detailed operational assessment in addition to the valuation report described in Project I. This will be completed in the place of the limited operational assessment as described in Project I and will encompass an in-depth review of all issues of the Practice. Appraiser will perform this assessment via an on-site review and will summarize—in detail—the findings of the analysis. Furthermore, Appraiser will summarize those areas of operations currently being completed in the Practice and identify any improvements that could be made and suggest any corrective action regarding the current operations.

The detailed assessment will include, but is not limited to, a review of the following operational areas:

- Personnel review
  - —Hours worked
  - —Pay scale
  - —Benefits
  - —Competence level
  - —Management structure
  - —Duties and job responsibilities
- Revenue cycle analyses (including billing/collections functions)

* These hours/fees are in addition to Project I, Phase III hours/fees.

FIGURE 8-1 Letter of Engagement (*continued*)

- Internal controls and procedures
- Management information/practice operating systems review
- Scheduling procedures
- Patient management/patient flow procedures
- Regulatory compliance
- Lease reviews
  —Facility leases
  —Capital leases
  —Employee leases
  —Equipment leases
- Expense structure
- Financial performance (historical and prospectively)
- Demographic analysis
  —Current patients' payer analysis
  —Current patients' age analysis
  —Current patients' zip code analysis

Professional Fees

Estimated hours to complete this phase: x to x hours @ $xxx per hour (one consultant)	$xxx to $xxx

Summary of Fees

Project I: Practice Valuation and Limited Assessment

Phase One:	Off-site preparation (x to x hours @ $xxx per hour)	$xxx to $xxx
Phase Two:	On-site review (x to x days on-site @ $xxx per day)	$xxx to $xxx
Phase Three:	Formal report (x to x hours @ $xxx per hour)	$xxx to $xxx
Total fees for Project I		**$xxx to $xxx**

Project II: Detailed Operational Assessment

Formal Report (x to x hours @ $xxx per hour)	$xxx to $xxx
Total fees for Project II (in addition to Project I fees)	**$xxx to $xxx**
Total Fees, Projects I and II	**$X,XXX to $X,XXX**

FIGURE 8-1 Letter of Engagement (*continued*)

Subsequent to completing the above phases, further needed analysis and assistance in the negotiation and the purchase/sale process as well as any other updates to the valuation, including changes of assumptions, etc, will be subject to additional professional fees. Unless agreed otherwise, Appraiser's fee of $xxx to $xxx per hour will prevail, depending upon the consultant's experience level. All work will be documented and substantiated by Appraiser, submitted to the Client.

An initial billing of $xxx toward the completion of this assignment will result at the execution of this Agreement. The remainder will be billed after the completion of each project. The Client will remit payment to Appraiser within 10 days of invoicing.

The Client will also reimburse Appraiser for its travel and out-of-pocket expenses incurred by its consultant(s) during this project. Appraiser will submit proper documentation to support these expenses. Such charges include, but are not limited to, airfare, lodging, meals, rental car, parking, etc, while onsite. Overnight shipping expenses will be reimbursed to Appraiser within thirty (30) days of billing.

Execution below indicates agreement to Appraiser to pursue the below-noted projects associated with the preparation and completion of this assignment.

Project(s) to Complete (By initialing, you signify your decision to complete the project.)

Project I: ____________________

Project II: ____________________

FOR ATLANTA ORTHOPEDIC PHYSICIANS, PA

____ ______________

John D. Smith, MD Date

____ ______________

Bob A. Jones, MD Date

FOR HEALTHCARE APPRAISERS, LLC

____ ______________

Consultant Date

The referenced practice and physician names in this and the following figures are, to the best of the author's knowledge, fictitious and not true practices/providers.

FIGURE 8-1 Letter of Engagement (*continued*)

valuation based on their knowledge as an appraiser. However, without a thorough understanding of the operations of these entities, it is highly unlikely that they would be able to perform a detailed assessment. This is why, especially in the area of medical practice, it is beneficial to procure a valuation professional with a detailed working knowledge of the field. Such a professional can often provide additional knowledge that another professional who is less familiar with practice operations may not.

Other Agreements

The appraiser may choose to incorporate these other agreements into the letter of engagement or may provide them as separate documents, as they are presented here. These documents provide additional support and representation for the client to the appraiser and vice versa. They also add a supplementary level of understanding. These documents include the following:

- *Confidentiality agreement.* This letter maintains that anything that is discussed between the client and the appraiser will remain confidential at all times, before, during, and after the valuation process. Although confidentiality is expected, this agreement further documents the understanding between the two parties. Figure 8-2 is an example of a confidentiality agreement.
- *Statement of independence.* The purpose of this statement is to ensure that the appraiser and the client and any other third parties shall remain independent at all times. Again, this should be self-evident; however, an official statement documenting the fact that the appraiser shall remain independent throughout this process and that no party shall attempt to impugn the appraiser's independence is necessary. Figure 8-3 is an example of a statement of independence.
- *Statement of undue influence.* The statement of undue influence is another document that should support that which should hold true in any situation. This statement documents the fact that the professional will not be influenced by any party and serves as proof for the appraiser's professionalism. Figure 8-4 provides an example that is not an agreement between all parties but rather a statement being made by the appraiser.
- *Medical records confidentiality agreement.* When valuing a medical practice, an appraiser must consider the patients' medical records. This information is highly confidential and should be treated as such. This is why it is appropriate to produce a confidentiality agreement noting the purpose for the appraiser examining the records, the limit on information that will be taken from each record, and the fact that the appraiser has received permission by the appropriate individuals to review these confidential

Confidentiality Agreement

Atlanta Orthopedic Physicians, PA, of Atlanta, Georgia, (the "Client") has agreed to engage Healthcare Appraisers, LLC (the "Appraiser") to perform a valuation and assessment of the operations of South Atlanta Physical Therapy, LLC (the "Practice").

The Client, Practice, and Appraiser acknowledge the sensitive and confidential nature of the information to be disclosed, and acknowledge the importance of the continued confidentiality of such information.

In consideration for consent to disclose this information, Appraiser agrees and covenants that it will not at any time, directly or indirectly, disclose or communicate to any person, firm, or corporation, in any manner whatsoever, any information disclosed to Appraiser without the express written consent of the Practice, understanding the report will go directly to the Practice and be available for its review and internal use.

FOR ATLANTA ORTHOPEDIC PHYSICIANS, PA

____________________________ ______________

Date

FOR SOUTH ATLANTA PHYSICAL THERAPY, LLC

____________________________ ______________

Date

FOR HEALTHCARE APPRAISERS, LLC

____________________________ ______________

Consultant Date

FIGURE 8-2 Confidentiality Agreement

Source: *Assessing the Value of the Medical Practice,* 2nd ed.

documents. When an appraiser is to take note of such important and confidential data, it is beneficial to all parties involved that a statement of confidentiality be executed. Individuals with access to protected health information are required to execute a business associate agreement under the Health Insurance Portability and Accountability Act (HIPAA; see Figure 8-5).

- *Privacy statement.* Every appraisal (and consultative) firm should have a statement documenting its privacy clause and the

Healthcare Appraisers, LLC (the "Appraiser") acknowledges that as the selected professional to perform the valuation and assessment of South Atlanta Physical Therapy, LLC (the "Practice"), it will perform its work with total independence and in no way will the value of the Practice be influenced by the entity that will pay the appraiser's professional fees (ie, the "Client").

Furthermore, Appraiser certifies that to the best of its knowledge, there exists no known conflicts of interest that would cause or even illicit the perception of a lack of independence pertaining to the valuation of the Practice.

FOR HEALTHCARE APPRAISERS, LLC

______________________________ ____________

Consultant Date

FIGURE 8-3 Statement of Independence

Source: *Assessing the Value of the Medical Practice,* 2nd ed.

Atlanta Orthopedic Physicians, PA (the "Client") has requested that Healthcare Appraisers, LLC (the "Appraiser") complete a valuation and assessment of South Atlanta Physical Therapy, LLC (the "Practice"). The Client acknowledges that Appraiser will function in total independence and therefore will not exert undue influence to in any way affect the findings and Appraiser's recommendations. The fee for this work will in no way be contingent upon the valuation total derived or the conclusions derived therein.

FOR ATLANTA ORTHOPEDIC PHYSICIANS, PA

______________________________ ____________

Date

FOR HEALTHCARE APPRAISERS, LLC

______________________________ ____________

Consultant Date

FIGURE 8-4 Statement of Undue Influence

Source: *Assessing the Value of the Medical Practice,* 2nd ed.

Atlanta Orthopedic Physicians, PA, of Atlanta, Georgia, (the "Practice") has agreed to engage Healthcare Appraisers, LLC, to perform a valuation and assessment of the operations of South Atlanta Physician Therapy, LLC (the "Practice").

The Client, Practice, and Appraiser acknowledge the sensitive and confidential nature of the information provided within medical records and the importance of such information. Under the Health Information Technology for Economic and Clinical Health Act (the "HITECH Act"), **Health Insurance Portability and Accountability Act** (HIPAA) privacy and security requirement, and in consideration for consent to disclose this information, Appraiser agrees and covenants that it will not at any time, directly or indirectly, disclose or communicate to any person, firm, or corporation, in any manner whatsoever, a patient's name or in any way jeopardize the privacy between the provider/physician and the patient. It is understood, however, that this review may encompass specific recommendations for improvements needed in documentation, adherence to risk management, protocols, including proper chart organization, all of which will be done within the context and purpose of Appraiser's review.

FOR ATLANTA ORTHOPEDIC PHYSICIANS, PA

______________________________ _______________

Date

FOR SOUTH ATLANTA PHYSICIAL THERAPY, LLC

______________________________ _______________

Date

FOR HEALTHCARE APPRAISERS, LLC

______________________________ _______________

Consultant Date

FIGURE 8-5 Medical Records Confidentiality Agreement (HIPAA Business Associate Agreement)

limits of its liability with regard to the privacy it provides to the client (and other third parties) and information pertaining to the client (and other third parties).

Appraisal Fee

The fee for the appraisal is one of the most important facets of the engagement both to the client and to the appraiser: to the appraiser because this serves as the method by which the respective firm will generate its revenues, and to the client because this will be the fund into which the client is responsible to pay for the services provided.

Often, the appraiser and the client have differing perspectives on appropriate professional fees. This is why it is imperative for the appraiser to outline the fees, terms of payment, and method of calculation.

Typically, a professional firm's fees are calculated and charged to the client by an hourly rate, and for each incremental time period (ie, either every quarter-hour, half-hour, or other fraction) of work provided. While larger firms and larger clients may be more amenable to such a fee structure, smaller practices/clients are typically very cost conscience and tend to shy away from such fee structures. In these cases, it may be appropriate (see Figure 8-1) for the appraiser to base fees on an hourly basis and cap the total fees of the project. This arrangement will ensure the client that the charges will not exceed those quoted in the letter of engagement.

However, the appraiser must be careful when quoting hourly based, capped fees. If the project becomes too extensive and requires more work than originally assumed to produce a suitable valuation, then the appraiser will likely absorb the cost of those additional hours that cannot be billed. Also, the client may request that additional work be completed or try to take advantage of the appraiser for work not included in the scope of the original letter of engagement. Thus, the appraiser should always include in the letter of engagement specific wording on what the valuation entails, and anything over and above that. Moreover, it should indicate that if information is discovered that considerably changes the time that the appraiser must contribute, then the extended time should be subject to additional fees. It may be difficult to distinguish what is and what is not a part of the original assignment; thus, it is beneficial to discuss this with the client before work begins.

Another method in which the appraiser may generate fees is to set a flat fee that the client is charged. While the client may favor this method, it often puts the burden of completing the project under the set fee on the appraiser. This cost structure may be suitable for smaller projects (eg, when a client chooses to request a brief, hypothetical valuation for internal analytical purposes); it is not generally the best method for larger, more substantial projects.

All of the previously stated methods are suitable for basing the professional fees for a project; however, some methods of basing fees are not appropriate. Most notably is the method of basing professional fees on a percentage of actual value. This method not only puts the client at a disadvantage, but it could also potentially impugn the independence and unduly influence the judgment of the appraiser by raising the valuation conclusion to increase the fees that are due. It is important for the appraiser to note that the fees from the project are not based on the conclusion as calculated in the appraisal. (Appraisal fees are discussed in more detail in Chapter 4.)

Conclusion

This chapter addresses many important steps of assessing the value of a health care entity that must be defined before the appraisal can be completed. Each aspect affects the integrity of the whole process, from the issue of what will be valued, to how it will be valued, to the details of the agreement, and the establishment of fees. The more precisely defined the assignment, the better the client's valuation.

Endnotes

1. American Society of Appraisers. Introduction to Business Valuation, Part 1. In: *Principles of Valuation: Business Valuation Student Manual, BV 201.* Herndon, VA: American Society of Appraisers; 2002:26–27.
2. Ibid, 14.
3. Internal Revenue Service. Revenue Ruling 59–60. Available at http://www.hantzmonwiebel.com/live_data/documents/ruling-59-60.pdf. Accessed June 10, 2011.
4. Pratt S, Reilly R, Schweihs R. *Valuing a Business: The Analysis and Appraisal of Closely Held Companies.* 4th ed. New York, NY: McGraw-Hill; 2000.
5. Ibid, 31.
6. American Society of Appraisers. General Requirements for Developing a Business Valuation. In: *Business Valuation Standards, BVS-I.* Herndon, VA: American Society of Appraisers; 2001.

CHAPTER 9 Valuation Methods

OUTLINE

I. Introduction
II. Market Approach
   A. Application of the Market Approach
   B. Market Approach Valuation Methodologies
   C. Normalization of the Financial Statements
   D. Calculation and Selection of Multiples
   E. Analyze, Compare, and Adjust Multiples
   F. Discounts and Premiums
      1. Calculate the Value
      2. Source of Market Data
   G. Market Approach Conclusion
III. Asset-based Approach
   A. Net Asset Value Method
      1. Tangible Asset Value
      2. Value in Use
      3. Liquidation Value
      4. Accounts Receivable
      5. Intangible Assets Value
      6. Liabilities
   B. Excess Earnings Method
   C. Asset-based Approach Conclusion
IV. Income Approach
   A. Pro Forma Financial Projections
      1. Growth Expectations
      2. Post-transaction Physician Compensation
      3. Expected Changes in Payer Payment

B. Discount Rates
  1. Build-up Method
  2. Capital Asset Pricing Model
C. Weighted Average Cost of Capital
D. Value Calculation
E. Reconciliation of Values and Conclusion of Value
V. Conclusion

Now that the foundation for the appraisal and valuation process has been explained, the various methodologies used for calculating the value of a health care entity (eg, a medical practice, ambulatory surgical center, business units that deliver health care) will be examined. Thus far, the three basic approaches of valuation have been defined as the following:

- Market approach
- Asset-based approach
- Income approach

All three approaches are acceptable to use in the appraisal process. Furthermore, Chapter 8 discusses the concept of tangible and intangible value and how it relates to the three approaches. In this chapter, each approach will be examined and reviewed in detail. (It should be noted that all figures in Chapter 9 are based on the financial statements found in Appendix B.)

Market Approach

The market approach uses comparative analysis of prices paid for similar assets or businesses in the marketplace. "This approach is based on the principle of substitution premise in that a prudent buyer will pay no more for property than it would cost to acquire a substitute property with the same utility."[1] While the process is different, this is similar in many respects to the "comparable sales" method used in real estate appraisal, whereas the subject company being valued (eg, the facility, house) is compared to prices paid to similar businesses (eg, facilities, buildings).

Application of the Market Approach

The market approach has the advantage of being easy to understand and apply. It does not require complicated financial projections and calculations; since it is based on valuation multiples indicated by comparable transactions, it reflects the current trends and expectations.

On the other hand, the market approach has its limitations in terms of applicability. The most common reason it cannot be applied in many small private medical practice valuations is that it is difficult to find comparable guideline practices. Moreover, the appropriate application of the market approach requires the appraiser to appropriately identify comparable transactions.

In applying the market approach, one must understand the basic principles underlying this valuation approach:

1. Comparability: In this process, the appraiser uses guideline companies, or similar companies, to derive multiples that are then applied to data from the health care entity or medical practice (ie, subject company) under consideration. Do not confuse the term guideline companies with *comparable companies* because rarely are two—much less three or four—entities so much alike that they can be considered comparable. In fact, the Internal Revenue Service (IRS) Revenue Ruling 59-60 (RR 59-60) defines the companies that should be used as *similar*. Generally, guideline companies should be in the same or at least in a very similar business as the subject company.

   In addition, size, growth expectation, and risks should also be examined to determine comparability. Typically, size can be measured via sales, total assets, or market capitalization.
2. Timeliness: Market transaction data that are used in the market approach must reflect the market condition consistent with the effective date of the valuation. In general, the guideline public company method should be established based on the transaction prices as of the valuation's effective date. In the guideline market transaction method, transactions must have occurred within a reasonable period of the effective date, typically less than three to five years. However, given the rapid changes of the health care market, this period can be shortened to a year or a few months.
3. Availability: To apply the market approach, it is essential that the price information of the market transaction is available. In addition, to ensure the appropriate application of the market multiples, the appraiser must also obtain sufficient quantitative and qualitative information about the guideline companies.

   Typically, minority transaction data for publicly traded companies are available from the stock market. Price and deal term information can also be obtained from Security and Exchange Commission (SEC) filings and databases such as Capital IQ.

   Another source of market transaction data is from merger and acquisition transactions involving closely held companies. This information can be found in SEC filings (if a business is acquired by a publicly traded company) or various deal databases. Unfortunately, detail and deal terms relative to closely held company transactions are typically incomplete and difficult to compare.

Market Approach Valuation Methodologies

There are two generally accepted valuation methodologies under the market approach. These include the guideline public company method and the merger and acquisition method.

The American Society of Appraiser's Business Valuation Standard defines the guideline public company method as "a method within the market approach whereby market multiples are derived from market prices of stocks of companies that are engaged in the same or similar line of business, and that are actively traded on a free and open market."[2]

Apparently, the guideline public company method relies on the relevant trading information that is readily available on the open stock market. Therefore, it has the advantage of having a great of deal of financial and operating data available, because publicly traded companies are required to disclose such information to stockholders and market regulators. Given the availability of information, timeliness can be easily achieved, as typically the appraiser is able to select transaction data on or close to the date of the valuation.

The other valuation methodology within the market approach is the merger and acquisition method or transaction method. This method uses the transaction multiples dictated by the merger and acquisition transactions that have taken place. Unlike the guideline public company method, which relies on price information of minority marketable shares, this method, in most cases, derives multiples based on control interest of a business. (Note: minority marketable shares refer to the actively traded noncontrolling interest stock price of public companies.)

When valuing the control interest of a stock that is very nonmarketable, this method is usually preferable. However, data from various transactions may be more difficult to find and discern due to the nonpublic nature of the transactions. Numerous firms gather these types of data, which would prove to be useful (see Appendix C).

The merger and acquisition method carries with it a number of advantages and disadvantages, although it is in the appraiser's judgment to determine if one outweighs the other. Some of the advantages include the following[3]:

- Can provide a reasonable indication of the prices at which entire entities/practices change hands
- Objective source of data
- Informed buyers and sellers

Some of the disadvantages include the following:

- Hard to find similar companies that have been acquired
- Hard to obtain actual terms relative to the acquisitions
- Hard to interpret the data and what exactly is being bought and sold
- May involve specific buyers that will pay a premium for special or unique considerations

Normalization of the Financial Statements

Once the guideline company(s) has been determined, both quantitative financial information and qualitative information of the subject company and the guideline companies must be compared. To ensure that the information is more relevant to the valuation, the appraiser must carefully review the financial statements of the subject company and the guideline companies and make the following adjustments:

1. Accounting method and policy: In cases in which the financial statements of the subject company and the guideline companies are prepared based on different accounting methods (for example, accrual vs cash accounting), adjustments must be made so that the financial statements can be comparable for analytical purposes.
2. Discretionary or nonoperating items: Medical practices, whether operated as a sole proprietorship or other legal entities, often include assets or expenses that are not typically found or required within the entities. These are referred to as *discretionary* or *nonoperating expenses.*

   For example, consider the case in which physician owners in a practice have historically been compensated considerably more (or less) than the norm for their specialty. This would, therefore, make it difficult to compare the practice's expenses to those of the guideline company. While this comparison is not considered illegal or unethical, it is something that must be addressed. To make a legitimate comparison, the appraiser must have the same underlying assumptions at both companies.

   Depending on the situation (particularly if it is a sole proprietorship or a smaller group practice), the physicians' compensation should be restated or not considered at all. Often, provider compensation will be considered as a *below the line* item from normal operating expenses.
3. Extraordinary/nonrecurring items: Furthermore, the appraiser must restate any *nonrecurring expenses.* These expenses are not regular deductions, such as rent, utilities, or employee compensation, but rather expenditures related to one-time occurrences. For

example, in a medical practice, these expenses may be associated with items such as a temporary increase in legal and consulting fees or a special charge due to expanding services. While this may be a legitimate expense, it is not something that is expected to occur on a regular basis. (Appraiser beware: Some organizations will classify some expenses as nonrecurring, such as a malpractice settlement or the lawyer fees pertaining to a malpractice case, which, in most instances, is fine. However, if it is noted that the practice, for example, has had charges pertaining to malpractice settlements and lawyer fees consistently throughout the review period and beyond, it may not be correct to just assume that these are nonrecurring.)

Calculation and Selection of Multiples

Once guideline companies have been identified and comparable data obtained, the information from the guideline companies should be used to calculate the multiples. As previously stated, in spite of the fact that a great deal of transaction, financial, and operational information is available from public companies, the appraiser must delve deeper into the guideline company's operations than simply applying the multiples to the subject company's metrics. "In fact, due to differences between companies, just a stock price for the guideline company will often prove useless. This is why we must calculate various multiples of the stock prices of the guideline companies in relation to such things as their earnings, cash flow, book value, etc."[4]

In general, there are two types of multiples: equity market multiples and invested capital market multiples. Equity multiples are applicable in the valuation of minority interest and/or when the capital structure of the subject and guideline companies are similar. On the other hand, invested capital multiples are applied in valuation of a control interest and/or situations in which there are significant differences in the capital structures of the subject and guideline companies. Using invested capital multiples allows for a comparison without adjusting for differing degrees of financial leverage, which can hinder using companies that are debt laden.

Some of the common multiples include the following:

- Equity Multiples
  - Market value of common equity (MVEq)/pretax earnings
  - MVEq/cash flow
  - MVEq/net income
- Invested Capital Multiples
  - Market value of invested capital (MVIC)/earnings before interest and taxes (EBIT)

- MVIC/earnings before interest, taxes, depreciation, and amortization (EBITDA)
- MVIC/sales

The selection of appropriate multiples to apply is subject to the professional judgment of the appraiser. "The appraiser must utilize both quantitative and qualitative analysis to choose the ratio (multiple) best suited to the subject company."[5]

Analyze, Compare, and Adjust Multiples

Once the multiples are calculated, it is important that the appraiser performs quantitative and qualitative analyses of the subject company and compares the corresponding characteristics of them with those of the guideline companies.

The guideline companies will likely differ in ways that cannot be determined by any figures, although certainly they may affect the inherent risk of the guideline company. Applicability of the multiples of these guideline companies should be measured by qualitative characteristics. A list of the qualitative features may include a number of variables; some of the more common include:

- Size
- Market share
- Geographic location
- Managed care population/reliance
- Services offered
- Provider and management depth, etc

Analyses and comparisons relative to quantitative characteristics, on the other hand, primarily focus on financial performance factors. The key objectives of this analysis are to determine the subject company's risk profile and investment outlook as compared with those of the guideline companies. While quantitative analyses usually use basic financial analysis techniques, including trend analysis and peer analysis, in the analysis for the market approach valuation, the appraiser typically pays special attention to the following key areas:

- Size (charges, payments, and total assets)
- Historical growth and growth perspective
- Capital structure
- Profitability

Discounts and Premiums

The multiples from both methods (ie, merger and acquisition method and public company method) provide excellent information on which to base the value of the subject company. It is important, however, that further adjustments are applied to the multiples to ensure that the multiples applied to the subject company's metrics appropriately reflect the desired level of value consistent with the purpose of the particular valuation.

Discounts and premiums applied in business valuations generally include those related to marketability and control.

As previously discussed, stock trading prices from publicly traded companies reflect the prices of minority, marketable shares. To apply such multiples to an appraisal of a majority interest of a large, privately held specialty medical practice, the appraisal should consider applying a control premium and a discount for lack of marketability.

It is likely that the controlling interest of an entity is worth more than a minority interest because with control comes the ability to make operations-altering decisions. A minority interest usually does not have such control. Furthermore, if minority interests are used to place multiples on a control valuation, it is likely that a premium will be placed on the guideline company's multiple to reflect the controlling interest.

Conversely, while a controlling interest may call for a premium on a guideline company's multiple, the fact that the company is closely held may require a discount to be applied. Although a controlling interest may mean that a single person may significantly determine the future of the company, this greatly affects that person's ability to buy and sell all or portions of the company or their marketability. However, a publicly owned company is easy to exchange and is one of the most liquid financial holdings.

Does this mean that the premium for controlling interest will cancel out the discount of lack of marketability? This situation occurs when the value of a knowledgeable appraiser can provide invaluable skill and advice.

There are no tables in which to find answers to the aforementioned situation. Certainly, the appraiser can examine past appraisals that are available to the public to help understand how previous discounts and premiums were applied and how they affected that appraiser's decisions. In addition, volumes of studies have been completed that try to address this matter. This process, however, is primarily a subjective one that will rely heavily on the assumptions and reasoning behind such applications and the application of these studies.

Calculate the Value

When the adjustments have been made and the appropriate multiples have been chosen, these are applied to the subject company's corresponding financial metrics so that a value indication can be calculated.

For example, the average market value of invested capital (MVIC) to revenue multiple for the guideline companies is 1.2. Multiply this ratio of IC to revenues by the subject company's revenues of $2,360,975, and a total value of $2,833,170 is calculated. However, because MVIC was used, the appropriate level of interest-bearing debt for the subject company must be subtracted to determine the equity value (ie, approximately $427,730). Before any discounts or premiums are considered, this amount would calculate a market value of equity (MVEq) of $2,405,440 based on the market multiple method.

If the MVEq to revenue multiple was used under the similar transaction method, the average for the guideline companies was 1.24. This amount would then be multiplied by the subject company's revenues of $2,360,975 to equal $2,927,609 (again, before the application of any discounts or premiums). However, because the MVIC was not used and this is only the value of the company's equity, debt does not have to be subtracted.

Based on this analysis, one can see that the values associated with the different ratios (multiples) will vary, although both cases are calculated before the application of any discounts or premiums. Depending on the value being sought and the market figures that are used, these discounts or premiums may considerably affect the value.

The market valuation and the application of various multiples have been considerably simplified for demonstration purposes. It is assumed that any quantitative and qualitative adjustments have already been made before any calculation of value commences. Also, in most cases, the most viable multiples may not be an average; valuation consultants must use their professional judgment in the selection and application of transaction multiples. Again, this process has been somewhat oversimplified for demonstration purposes.

Source of Market Data

To perform a viable market analysis of a company, necessary data must be available to perform the analysis. Appendix C provides numerous resources from which an appraiser of a business could obtain a large amount of information.

As discussed, stock prices and financial information relative to public companies are readily available via a variety of sources. This information can be easily obtained from the public companies' quarterly and annual filings as well as the stock market.

Despite the availability of public company data, many times it is very difficult to apply the guideline public company method in valuations of small medical practices simply because there are very few, if any, publicly traded medical groups. Most often, the guideline public company method is widely used in valuations of hospitals, ambulatory surgery centers, and imaging centers.

The merger and acquisition method relies on pricing multiples derived from comparable transactions that have taken place. A number of databases commonly use appraisals for the research of transaction information. These include Bloomberg, Capital IQ, Done Deals, Mid Market Comps, Mergerstat, **BIZCOMPS**®, and Pratt's Stats®. In addition, Goodwill Registry and Irving Levin Associates, Inc, provide special health care transaction data.

It is important to note that definitions of transaction terms often vary from database to database, making it very difficult to use returns from multiple databases. Therefore, it is imperative that appraisers carefully review the instructions when using each database and analyze each transaction carefully.

Market Approach Conclusion

The market approach most often requires an investment of a large amount of research and time to accurately calculate the applied multiples to the subject company. This method also requires a great deal of subjectivity when determining how to apply the various multiples that are calculated. Moreover, while it may not be the best for smaller, closely held medical practices (eg, a solo practitioner), it is an indispensable method that should certainly be considered in valuations of all sizes.

Asset-based Approach

The asset-based approach uses a number of different methods to value both tangible and intangible assets.

This approach is often used to value an entity that is going out of business or discontinuing operations; it is less frequently used as a supporting valuation of a going concern. Many experts share the idea that the asset-based approach is not best suited for service companies (eg, a medical practice) or to value the intangible assets of a company. However, in cases in which the market approach is not applicable and the income approach (discussed later) calculates a negative value, this may be the only method in which any value can be applied to an entity. In this case, it is perfectly acceptable.

Net Asset Value Method

Net asset value method values an entity by assessing the economic value of the assets on the balance sheet and subtracting the value of its liabilities. While this method appears to be as easy as adding all of the assets from the balance sheet to determine the value, it is not quite that simple. Actually, an appraiser must complete a considerable amount of analysis to determine the correct number associated with each of the asset categories. To do this, the appraiser must determine the adjusted book value of each of the asset categories.

Generally, the best place to determine an entity's assets is from the balance sheet. However, most medical practices—especially smaller ones—pay little, if any, attention to the balance sheet (as opposed to a larger entity, whose balance sheet is a key financial management tool and, therefore, maintained actively). This is because most medical practices complete their accounting on a cash basis (or a modified cash basis), thus making the balance sheet somewhat inaccurate.

Tangible Asset Value

In Chapter 7, tangible assets were defined, and several examples were presented. Tangible assets consist of physical items, such as equipment, furniture, supplies, fixtures, cash, accounts receivable, and inventory. For purposes of this review, tangible assets are limited only to equipment, furniture, and the like.

For accounting purposes, most of these tangible assets have a depreciable value that is reduced over a specific period of time—usually over a period of years—depending on the type of assets and method of depreciation used. For tax purposes, most practices choose to use the accelerated depreciation method, thus making the net book value (ie, original cost minus accumulated depreciation) of the tangible assets greater than their actual fair market value. For example, if a medical practice purchases an examination table, and depreciates that table over a period of five years without residual value, at the end of that five-year period that examination table will be fully depreciated and it will have no book value. However, this does not mean that the practice would just give this table away for free because it has no book value. This process exemplifies why book value may not be the best method of valuing tangible assets. The following are a number of definitions used in valuing tangible assets:

- Reproduction cost new: The cost of reproducing a new replica of an item on the basis of current prices with the same or closely similar materials
- Replacement cost new: The current cost of a similar new item having the nearest equivalent utility as the item being appraised
- Depreciated replacement cost new: Replacement cost new less depreciation
- Fair market value in continued use (value in use): The fair market value of an item based on its original purchase price and the continued utilization of the item in conjunction with all other installed items
- Liquidation value: Amount expected by the immediate sale of the assets, including orderly liquidation and forced liquidation

For purposes of valuing a medical practice, the appraiser most often will be concerned with only the value in use and the liquidation value.

Value in Use

The definition of value in use is applied when valuing a practice under the premise of continued use. Under this premise, the furniture and equipment are valued as a part of an income-producing business enterprise, meaning that they have greater value to the purchaser of the practice because they are "in use" and play a part in the generation of revenue to the practice, as opposed to buying the assets in "piecemeal" fashion.

The valuation of tangible assets typically starts with a detailed inventory of the practice's assets. During the process, the appraiser can make a detailed list of the assets and value each one individually. However, in medium to larger entities this would likely be impossible. In this case, the appraiser may have to combine the different items per the tangible asset inventory from the entity's federal tax returns (an excellent place to get information such as number of and original purchase price of the entity's assets) and organize them by category. Often, the appraiser will also rely on the assistance of the practice management and obtain verification and confirmation of the accuracy of the asset inventory.

The cost approach and the market approach are typically used for valuing tangible assets. The starting point for valuation of used equipment is generally set with its "replacement cost new" basis, considering the current market cost of a similar item with equivalent utility.

While this approach may seem fairly straightforward, it may not be so easy to determine the asset's replacement cost of a similar new item. If the entity, or practice in this case, has kept good records over the years, then it should have the original cost of the items, although this is frequently not the case. In fact, most medical practices, especially smaller ones, typically keep poor records of these items. If the entity cannot provide these documents, the appraiser must determine the approximate cost of the items.

This process can be difficult for the appraiser because of the extent to which items differ. Medical equipment is generally easier because it is highly identifiable (eg, a Ritter 104 examination table, a General Electric x-ray machine). Office equipment, on the other hand, can be more difficult to determine. For example, without a thorough inspection—likely by someone familiar with furniture construction—it would be difficult to determine if a physician's executive desk set is custom-made mahogany or a manufactured set made to look custom made. Again, the appraiser has to use good judgment and determine what a correct price is.

Based on this information, the valuation consultant applies certain discounts by taking a number of issues into consideration, such as the ability to purchase all of the equipment at one time rather than having to find each item individually and determine the type of equipment, the usability of the equipment in its current position, and, most importantly, the condition of the equipment.

While there are some standards as to the percentage that is applied, based primarily on its condition and usability, there are no finite determinations as to the calculation of these percentages. As noted throughout the valuation process, the appraiser uses a great deal of subjectivity.

One reason why these are purely suggestions rather than standards is that these percentages truly vary from item to item based on a wide range of issues. For instance, consider a computer system that was purchased 18 months ago and is in excellent condition. A discount percentage of 70% to 80% could be applied. Technology—such as computers, printers, and fax machines—typically retains less value than other equipment because of its obsolescence rate. For this reason, the subjectivity that must be applied to calculate this percentage becomes apparent.

In determining the discount percentages, an appraiser should also take into consideration the age of the item and the fact that an item bought 30 years ago would almost certainly have cost less than an item bought within the last few years. Although, it is possible for an appraiser to apply the same cost to the same items, say for example, examination tables. This discount in price, however, is built into the in-place percentage. Regardless of the method used by the appraiser, it is essential that all assumptions within the report be clearly and consistently stated.

Once the discount percentage that will be applied to the item has been determined, the item's value can be calculated. To do this, the discount percentage is multiplied by the item's replacement cost of a new item.

Liquidation Value

If an entity's assets are being valued in use as a going concern and for future use in that going concern, then liquidation value can be seen as just the opposite. *Liquidation value* is the value of the assets of an entity that will close or not continue as a going concern.

Typically, when one hears the term *liquidation*, a hardship is implied. This, however, is not always the case. For example, an entity that chooses to discontinue business for no specific reason ceases operations as an ongoing entity. Before the entity can be fully dissolved, it must dispose of all of its tangible (as well as intangible) assets. In this case, an appraiser would assign the assets an *orderly liquidation value.* "That is the proceeds that one could expect from the sale of the assets held under normal conditions given a reasonable period of time in which to find a purchaser and sell the assets 'as is, where is,' with the purchaser assuming the cost of all removal and other related costs."[6]

The other type of liquidation, *forced liquidation*, occurs when a company must liquidate assets for the purpose of quickly offloading assets (whether the majority or a portion of the assets) for one reason or another. Usually, forced liquidation occurs when there is no time to find a purchaser. This situation could arise for a number of reasons. For example, a company may be forced to liquidate some of its assets to cover a short-term debt that has come due or to close out a facility as dictated by a landlord. This is often referred to as a *fire sale.*

The difference between the two types of liquidations is essentially the time involved. In one instance, an entity has unlimited time to find a willing buyer; in the other, it does not.

Both the forced liquidation and the orderly liquidation can be calculated in the same manner as the value in use discussed. However, with liquidations, some further discounts are applied. Typically, the orderly liquidation method will have a minimal discount applied to it, likely around 15% to 20%. This discount takes into account that purchasers are buying as is, where is, and that they will incur more costs due to moving and storage fees (that would not be incurred if the assets were going to be used in the same place and for the same reason).

Forced liquidation, on the other hand, will usually command much more of a discount to the in-place percentage. In the situation of a fire sale, or forced liquidation, a discount of 50% to 65% will be incurred, depending on the situation and the item.

Accounts Receivable

For most medical practice valuations, one asset item that will almost always need to be restated is that of patient accounts receivable (A/R). Because the majority of medical practices use a cash basis of accounting, A/R is typically not reflected on the balance sheet. Even if a practice does record A/R on its books, the book value of A/R is almost always not that which will actually be collected. To accurately measure the fair market value of A/R, an appraiser must consider the estimated collectable amount of the A/R based on additional factors including payer mix, payer contracting, and aging of the A/R. In fact, valuing A/R could entail a whole chapter of this book, if not an entire book itself. For purposes of this analysis, a company's A/R book value will be more than that which is actually collectable (often referred to as *fair collectable value*).

Intangible Assets Value

While the tangible assets are reflected in the entity's balance sheet, the intangible assets are off the balance sheet. Because balance sheets are indicative of an entity's cost-based assets, it is typical that intangible assets (often those that represent the most valuable assets) are not recorded. For valuation purposes, however, it is important that they are identified and valued.

For medical practices, generally intangible assets include assembled and trained workforce, negotiated contracts, established corporate operational infrastructure, trademark, brand names, and market share. To value these, a typical approach is to consider the recreation costs of these items.

It is important to note that the value of intangible assets does not necessarily exist in all medical practices. Generally, for intangible asset value to exist, it must be supported by positive net cash flows under the income approach (discussed in the next section). It is inappropriate to assign substantial value to intangible assets, such as workforce in place, when the income approach exhibits a value that is lower than the fair market value (FMV) of the practice's tangible assets.

Liabilities

Liabilities should also be taken into consideration in the application of the net asset value method. Liabilities under consideration for valuation purposes are generally interest-bearing long-term debts. As with tangible assets, FMV of liabilities does not always equal its book value. A typical method to value the FMV of liabilities is to calculate the sum of the liabilities' present value of future cash outflow, based on the discount rate as of the effective date of the valuation.

Excess Earnings Method

The excess earnings method, or formula method, is derived from IRS RR 68-609. This method attempts to value the intangible assets by considering appropriate returns on both tangible and intangible assets. Under most circumstances, normalized historical operating results would be used; however, if it is deemed appropriate by the analyst, recent operating results can be substituted.

This methodology is fairly straightforward, although, as has occurred in the past, the appraiser must make certain projections that are very subjective. In this case, the appraiser must determine the correct rate of return and capitalization rate. Ultimately, the best way to support all subjective figures is still through a thorough documentation of the underlying assumptions.

The following describes some simple procedures used to calculate the value:

Step 1: The appraiser must determine the market value of tangible assets and the normalized level of income.

a. The methods used to determine an entity's tangible asset value have been discussed previously in this chapter. The value determined by the appraiser by the appropriate standard of value will be applied here.

b. The appraiser must determine the appropriate level of earnings. The appraiser must determine whether to use normalized or actual earnings. Also, the appraiser must determine the appropriate time frame that is being considered. The basic premise behind this model is that it relies on historic information.

Step 2: This step is done to determine the level of excess earnings. It is conducted in the following parts:

a. First, the appraiser must determine an appropriate rate of return on the tangible assets (see Step 1.a). This will usually be similar to the entity's stated cost of capital. In the case of smaller companies, which may not know their internal cost of capital, it could be estimated by the analyst. This rate of return is then multiplied by the asset total to determine the excess earnings attributable to the company's net tangible assets.

b. Second, the appraiser will subtract this amount from the normalized net income (see Step 1.b) to obtain the excess earnings for the company.

Step 3: This step determines the actual intangible value attributable to the entity. This is done by capitalizing the excess earnings by an appropriate capitalization rate (discount rate minus long-term growth).

Step 4: The appraiser will add the intangible value (see Step 3) and the tangible value (see Step 2) to provide the total value of the entity.

While these steps are generally accepted as the traditional formula approach, various other methodologies have been used under this approach. This method provides an accurate approach to valuing an entity, but it only considers the company's historical operations, which is helpful but not what one wants when trying to determine the ongoing value of a company.

Asset-based Approach Conclusion

The ways in which to value not only a practice's actual tangible assets but also the practice's intangible assets are numerous. One must bear in mind that when calculating both the tangible and intangible assets via the two methodologies, the two figures must be combined to determine the total value of the entity.

Due to the many pitfalls associated with this approach, Business Valuation Standards (BVS) III specifies that "the asset approach should not be the sole appraisal approach used in assignment relating operating companies appraised as going concerns unless this approach is customarily used by sellers and buyers. In such cases, the appraiser must support the selection of this approach."[7]

While these methodologies may not suit entities such as medical practices, they can provide good benchmarks or supporting documentation. Although, in cases in which the entity exhibits no intangible value via the discounted cash flow methodology, the value of the entity's assets may be its only value. For this reason, calculations should virtually always be completed.

Income Approach

The income approach is the most widely accepted valuation approach for the valuation of medical practices. The discounted cash flow (DCF) method within the approach calculates the practice value based on the present value of its expected future economic benefit streams (ie, cash flows). The attraction of this method is that it considers the past operations and financial performance of an entity, then uses these figures in combination with the best estimates of future performance to place the value of the company.

As accepted and important as this methodology is, it requires more subjectivity from the analyst than any other approach. To appropriately establish the DCF calculations, an appraiser must have a good understanding of the subject company's past and prospective operations and financial performance. Also very important, the appraiser must rely on a thorough knowledge of the business being valued, the industry in which it competes, as well as the underlying assumptions used in the DCF methodology. Given the unique nature of the health care industry, industry-specific expertise is particularly important for medical practice valuations.

This section of the chapter provides an overview of the DCF methodology under the income approach and details that which is necessary to calculate the value of an entity under this approach. This chapter, however, will not serve as a "mini-MBA" in finance, detailing the minutiae and details that form the foundational information that has been developed over the years. The information used to develop this methodology has been spurred by some of the greatest minds to address the subject of finance, economics, accounting, and mathematics and fills volumes and volumes of books.

A lack of focus on this detail does not imply that this information is not significant, rather just the opposite; this methodology requires a detailed understanding of both financial theory and operations. Without such a basis, it would be impossible for anyone to be able to properly use the information that will be outlined in this section. Thus, it is assumed that the reader has a general understanding of finance, economics, mathematics, and accounting (among others) so that the aspects of this model are not only properly understood but also properly applied.

If one has a proper understanding of the theory underlying DCF methodology, then that approach can be applied to any company. The DCF methodology discussed in this book focuses on the valuation of a physician's practice and other health care entities. As such, some of the techniques used to value a medical practice may not be best suited for valuing other companies in other industries.

Pro Forma Financial Projections

The DCF method relies on appropriate and realistic projections of the practice's future cash flows. This method involves a detailed financial pro forma analysis, typically for five to seven years, based on the appraiser's professional judgment. The basis of the forecasts and assumptions applied in the DCF method should be reasonable and defensible based on the historical and market data available.

In the Instruction Program Textbook, the IRS expresses strong preference for the DCF method.[8] The most prominent advantage of the DCF model is that it allows the appraiser to take into consideration a variety of key factors that determine the value of a practice. Following in the next section are explanations of these key factors.

Growth expectations

Growth expectations relate to the practice's future earning capacity, the providers' ability to grow, and expected changes in the provider base (ie, type, number, and full-time status of physicians). For two practices with the same current earning levels and risks, the one that is expected to grow more has a higher value.

In general, the practice's historical track record provides the best indication of its future performance. To support its pro forma assumptions, it is essential that the appraiser completes an extensive analysis of the practice's historical productivity data and thoroughly documents how this affects the value; the most widely used financial analysis techniques include trending, benchmarking, and ratio analysis.

Post-transaction Physician Compensation

For most medical practices, physician compensation is the single largest expense item, representing between 20% and 50% of the medical revenue. Since the post-transaction compensation is a key component of the remuneration received by physician shareholders, it plays a crucial role in the determination of the practice value.

The FMV valuation of the practice sets forth the upfront purchase price of the practice. It measures the future economic benefits (after physician compensation is paid) to be received by any willing buyer of the practice. Subsequent to the transaction, the physician shareholders, as employees of the hospital, take away a portion of the future cash flows to be received by the buyers. As a result, the amount of post-transaction physician compensation has an inverse relationship to the practice value (ie, upfront purchase price). That is, the greater the post-transaction physician compensation, the lower the practice value.

To accurately measure the practice's FMV, it is critical that the pro forma and DCF calculations reflect the actual physician compensation plan to be provided to the physician owners post-transaction. Various fringe benefits, which are considered a component of the physician compensation, must also be applied. In instances in which a specific compensation plan is not available at the time the valuation is performed, the appraiser will apply an estimated FMV compensation amount for the initial valuation and conduct a "true up" of the valuation when the actual compensation becomes available.

Expected Changes in Payer Payment

In most cases, medical practices rely heavily on third-party payment. Changes in payer payment have a large impact on medical practice value. Therefore, it is imperative that the practice valuation takes into consideration the expected payment changes. This places great importance on retaining an experienced health care business appraiser who is able to skillfully and accurately determine the impact of future payment changes on the practice value.

Discount Rates

In its most basic form, the DCF method can be broken down into two parts, the return and the rate that will be used to capitalize the return. "A present value discount rate is an 'opportunity cost,' that is, the expected rate of return...that an investor would have to give up by investing in the subject investment—instead of available alternative investments that are comparable in terms of risk and other investments characteristics."[9]

Discount rate is a reflection of required rate of return. It is a measurement of risk, that is, the degree of uncertainty related to the realization of the expected future cash flows. There is a positive relationship between risk and required rate of return—the greater the perceived risk involved in an investment, the higher the required rate of return (discount rate).

Nevertheless, value has a negative relationship with discount rate. The higher the discount rate, the lower the value.

The selection of appropriate discount rate must be based on the types of values that the appraiser will measure. For the valuation of enterprise value (EV), or value of invested capital (EIC), the appraiser must use the weighted average cost of capital (WACC) as the discount rate for the cash flows. This is because EV/EIC is an economic measure reflecting the value pertaining to the entire business entity. Thus, the business' risk related to both equity and debt must be taken into consideration. On the other hand, required rate of return of equity should be used in valuing a practice's equity value.

Build-up Method

One of the most widely used methods for estimating the equity discount rate is the build-up method. It considers the required return of equity of a business based on the sum of a number of identifiable risk factors.

Under this method, equity discount rate is calculated based on the following formula:

$$R_e = R_f + ERP + SP +/- IRP + CSRP$$

Where:

R_e: Equity discount rate.

R_f: Risk-free rate of return. This usually is estimated based on long-term treasury rates (eg, treasury bonds having maturity of 10 to 30 years).

ERP: Risk premium for the "market." It is often estimated by using historical realized return or forward-looking estimates. A common source of the historical realized ERP is the *Stock, Bonds, Bills, and Inflation Classic Yearbook* (Ibbotson® SBBI®) published by Morningstar, Inc.

SP: Risk premium for size. Many researchers indicate that, in general, the smaller the company, the higher the required rate of return. Two frequently used sources of empirical data for the size premium are the SBBI and the *Duff & Phelps Risk Premium Report*.

IRP: Industry risk premium.

CSRP: Company-specific risk premium.

Capital Asset Pricing Model

Another frequently used approach to determine the return of equity is the capital asset pricing model (CAPM). This model was originally developed in the context of portfolio theory. This model can be exhibited as follows:

$$R_e = R_{rf} + \text{Beta}\ (R_m - R_{rf}) + Alpha$$

Where:

R_e: Expected rate of return, required rate of return, or the discount rate. This is the rate that is being calculated.

R_{rf}: Risk-free rate. This rate is associated with an investment that has no risk. (Absolutely no one thing has no risk; however, for purposes of this process, this rate will be referred to as *risk free.*) This rate of return is usually associated with an investment instrument such as US Treasury obligations. This risk-free rate can be found in any number of financial journals.

Beta: Measure of systematic risk. The simple definition of beta is the risk of the investment (or a similar investment) compared to the risk of the market. The market as a whole has a beta of 1.0, and the risk of the company is based on this standard. Therefore, an investment that has a beta of 0.8 would be considered less risky than the market. Correspondingly, an investment with a beta of 1.2 would be considered more risky than the market. (In some instances, a company may exhibit a beta of a negative number. In this case, the beta is counter-cyclical to the market.)

When there are enough comparables to perform a market analysis, the beta for the subject company may be derived from these sources (eg, the median beta for all guideline companies), such as Standard & Poor's Capital IQ Compustat[10]; however, if it has been determined that there are not enough market comparables to perform a market analysis, it may be appropriate to use the information provided by Ibbotson's *Stocks, Bonds, Bills & Inflation,* [11] which will provide a market beta.

$R_m - R_{rf}$: Equity risk premium. This premium is the level of risk that an investor can expect over and above the risk-free premium. This is the amount that an investor must be paid to invest money in another investment other than a risk-free investment. The figures used to calculate the equity risk premium are usually determined from Ibbotson's *Stocks, Bonds, Bills & Inflation.*[11]

Alpha: The measure of unsystematic risk in the market. While beta measures the systematic risk pertaining to an investment, alpha looks at more company- and market-specific data including size, specific market risks, and others.

Weighted Average Cost of Capital

The WACC is a blended discount rate that reflects the required rate of return to all financing sources, including both debt and equity, of the subject company.

The formula used to calculate a firm's WACC is as follows:

$$\text{WACC} = (k_e \times W_e) + (k_d\ [1 - t] \times W_d)$$

Where:

k_e: The firm's cost of equity

k_d: The firm's cost of debt

W_e: The percentage of equity, at market value

W_d: The percentage of debt capital (interest bearing debt), at market value

t: Effective tax rate

In the valuation of a controlling ownership interest, appraisers typically use the optimal capital structure, as opposed to the practice's actual capital structure, to calculate WACC. This is because (1) in most cases, the practice's excess earnings are retained by the owners, therefore making it very difficult to measure the practice's actual structure; and (2) acquirers of a controlling ownership interest have the ability to adjust the practice's capital structure post-acquisition.

Value Calculation

The DCF method is typically structured based on a five-year projection of the practice's future performance. Now that an appropriate rate of return has been determined, this can be applied to the projected cash flows to calculate the value of the interest. The basic DCF formula is as follows:

$$PV = \overbrace{\sum_{i=0}^{n} CFi / (1 + R)^n}^{\text{Discrete Cash Flows}} + \overbrace{\{[CF_{i+1} / (1 + g)] / (R - g)\} / (1+R)^n}^{\text{Terminal Value}}$$

Where:

CF_1 through CF_n: Projected cash flows (to invested capital or to equity)

R: Discount rate (WACC or equity rate of return)

n: Number of projected discrete cash flow periods

g: Long-term growth rate

$(R - g)$: Capitalization rate

Reconciliation of Values and Conclusion of Value

The final steps in a valuation are to reconcile the results from various valuation approaches and derive a conclusion of the practice's value.

If market approach and income approach are applied appropriately, values from these two approaches are generally close to each other. If not, a common cause would be inconsistent and unreasonable assumptions, lack of comparable transactions, or sometimes, computational errors. When this disparity happens, the appraiser should review the calculation and analysis that have been completed and verify the appropriateness and accuracy of each valuation step. For medical practice valuations, due to the lack of comparable public companies and comparable transactions, in many cases only the income approach is applied. However, the market approach is sometime used as a reality check.

To derive the conclusion of a valuation, appraisers must use their professional judgment by relying on a single valuation approach or multiple approaches.

Conclusion

The heart of this valuation process is the actual computation of the value. Numerous methodologies can be used to calculate the value of a medical practice or other entity, and the importance of a competent appraiser is stressed throughout.

Although various methodologies to value an entity can be employed, the knowledge of the appraiser and the standard of value that is being sought will dictate which basis of value to apply. The income approach is the one most recognized by the IRS; however, in certain situations, this may or may not be applicable (eg, a company that has no intangible value or a company that has invested a large amount of funds in real equipment).

The information that could have been conveyed in this chapter is vast, especially if the focus had not been primarily on medical entities. To provide a better understanding of the key methodologies and the processes by which they are calculated, much of the detail on which these methodologies are based (especially in the income methodology) has been avoided. Every detail regarding business valuation has not been covered; instead, a general understanding and insight into what comprises a medical entity valuation has been provided.

Endnotes

1. American Society of Appraisers. *Business Valuation Standards.* Herndon, VA: American Society of Appraisers; 2005:26.
2. American Society of Appraisers. Introduction to Business Valuation, Part 3. In: *The Market Approach to Value, BV 203.* Herndon, VA: American Society of Appraisers; 2008:101.
3. American Society of Appraisers. Introduction to Business Valuation, Part 1. In: *Principles of Valuation: Business Valuation Student Manual, BV 201.* Herndon, VA: American Society of Appraisers; 2002:67.
4. Ibid, 66.
5. Ibid, 75.
6. Ibid, 92.

7. American Society of Appraisers. *Business Valuation Standards.* Herndon, VA: American Society of Appraisers; 2002: 9.
8. Kaiser CF, Henchey A. *Instruction Program Textbook: Q. Valuation of Medical Practices.* 1996 Exempt Organization CPE Text. Available at http://www.irs.gov/pub/irs-tege/eotopicq96.pdf. Accessed June 17, 2011.
9. American Society of Appraisers. Introduction to Business Valuation, Part 1. In: *Principles of Valuation: Business Valuation Student Manual, BV 201.* Herndon, VA: American Society of Appraisers; 2002:159.
10. Www.compustat.com.
11. Www.morningstar.com.

CHAPTER 10 Valuation Guidelines

OUTLINE

I. Introduction
II. Multiples, Ratios, and Rules of Thumb
III. Application of Valuation Methodologies
IV. Research Through the Internet
V. Operations Assessment
VI. Valuation Data Checklist
VII. Conclusion

The previous chapters have reviewed the basic concepts of valuing health care facilities, the valuation process, and the specific methodologies used. This chapter addresses some of the relevant extraneous items, as well as the role of research and operations within the valuation process. Also included is a valuation checklist, which is a critical and useful tool to ensure that the appraiser is working with the essential information to reach a relevant valuation of the entity.

Multiples, Ratios, and Rules of Thumb

Multiples and ratios are integral to the valuation process. Two of the most important factors in the income approach are multiples, which include the capitalization rate and the discount rate. Some of the key financial benchmarks that are applied to a valuation are ratios, such as the debt ratio and current ratio, among others. Financial evaluation of a business requires a full appreciation and comprehension of multiples and ratios.

Rules of thumb provide another ratio that is often used in conducting valuations. *Rules of thumb* are industry standards expressed as a ratio of a specific number. For a medical practice, this ratio could be the number of active patients to net collections or active charts to net collections. For the most part, these ratios are useful to compare one entity to the subject entity, as is done using the market approach.

The problem with strictly using ratios in any particular analysis is that looking only at the ratio provides an inadequate context with regard to the entities being compared. What if the rules of thumb are taken from a random group of practices and no consideration is given to qualitative factors (such as the type and size) or details related to the practice? What if the practices are in an area that has a high level of capitated patients? This latter situation would likely result in a high number of active patients with only average income; the ratio being used would be the number of active patients to total collections. Furthermore, what if the ratios consist of only highly specialized practices in which active patients will be relatively low and collections should be relatively high?

These are all relevant questions that a valuator must ask when applying a certain type of ratio or rules of thumb to any analyses. Moreover, these are good illustrations as to why it is so critical that a valuator working with health care entities must be experienced and well-versed with the nuances of different types of health care facilities, and understand why and how they are different from businesses in other types of industries. A valuator also must understand the different types of facilities within the industry, because when comparing two medical practices that may be similar in size and services, there could still be significant differences that will skew various ratios due to variables, such as market demographics, reimbursement trends, and managed care statistics.

Ratios and multiples play an important role in the valuation process, but they must be applied in the appropriate context and with consideration. Rules of thumb are nothing more than blind ratios that can cause more problems if not applied accurately and appropriately, and in an applicable context to the subject of the valuation.

In many cases, people less familiar with the valuation process will make comments such as, "Can I just apply a multiple to find the value?" or "I talked to another practice administrator in [another part of the country] and their practice's value was based on a 1x multiple of revenue." They question why it takes so long to determine a practice's value when they believe they can gather a few multiples from the Internet or casual discussion at conferences, briefly review the income statement, make some calculations, apply the multiple, and arrive at a value.

Often, clients will make comments like, "I heard that medical practices are selling at six times income," and will wonder why their practice's value is so low. This is a common misconception that appraisers have to fight, and the onus will be on the appraiser to educate the client on what is appropriate. Multiples and ratios have their place in the valuation process but they are not always sufficient rules of thumb.

Application of Valuation Methodologies

Chapters 7 and 9 review a number of the standard valuation methodologies that are typically applied to determine the value of a medical entity. In the case of valuation, each project should be considered in its own right and the appropriate standard should be applied.

Accordingly, the appraiser should be knowledgeable in all fields of valuation science and know which methodology and standard should be applied and when it should be applied. This expertise is especially critical when valuations in the health care field can have far-reaching implications. Because of the role that the government plays in health care, a great deal of attention is paid to transactions that take place. This situation also arises due to the high preponderance of not-for-profit entities that exist in the health care marketplace. The government plays a much more active role in oversight of transactions involving health care facilities, particularly those involving not-for-profit entities, because these entities receive significant financial benefits in terms of taxes and managed care contracting.

An appraiser should be familiar with these nuances and know how they can potentially affect the valuation and any transfer of ownership. For instance, if a hospital is purchasing a medical practice, it is not appropriate to include the revenue generated by the practitioners for the hospital and compensate them directly for that revenue. That would violate any number of laws related to Stark and anti-kickback statutes (see Chapter 12). As such, a valuation methodology that considers this revenue may be inappropriate in this instance; an appraiser should be aware of this situation.

Another example of valuation assumptions in the instance of a health care facility transaction is the calculation of synergies. Both for-profit and not-for-profit health care facilities must go through a stringent regulatory approval process prior to a transaction closing. Although this process is typically more involved for not-for-profit entities, it is becoming a greater consideration for deals involving for-profit facilities, as clinical integration is increasing consolidation among hospitals and health systems with medical practices and outpatient/alternate site facilities, such as surgery centers, imaging centers, infusion centers, and vascular centers.

Thus, the overall volume of transactions is increasing, as well as the value attributed to many of these transactions. As such, the regulatory requirements, such as Hart-Scott-Rodino Antitrust Improvements Act of 1976, which apply to transactions valued at $150 million and higher, are becoming relevant to more and more transactions, as many medical groups in today's environment are exceeding this value threshold. Within these considerations, a valuator must understand what assumptions are appropriate in deriving a valuation that incorporates synergies, to ensure that no anti-trust concerns are related to those assumptions. Regulators have rejected many large transactions involving major not-for-profit health systems because of the valuation not being compliant with all of the relevant laws and statutes that govern such deals; this is not a position that an appraiser wants to encounter.

In general, health care entities can be highly dynamic and very unstable, and this is even more the case in small practices. Physicians and staff come and go and, in most markets, there is high portability for patients between providers (some health maintenance organizations in which patients are limited by who they can and cannot see may actually benefit the provider). All of these factors must be considered in the valuation process. This is why the entity should be valued for its future operations, not its past.

The market approach is a highly regarded method for valuing organizations, but should a practice receive a multiple of three times collections if two physicians have just left and there is no plan to replace them? If those collections cannot be assured in the future, why should the multiple be applied to them?

This is another reason why historical valuation methodologies, such as the asset-based approach to valuation, are sometimes unreliable. They consider the historical operations rather than the future operations. With the rapidly changing health care industry, how can these methods of valuation be applicable when they only look at the past and not the future?

In the past, many appraisers would rely on the replacement methodology for valuing the goodwill (ie, the intangible portion) of medical practices. Chapters 1 and 4 provide an in-depth description of this valuation methodology; essentially, it considers the price that it would take to "recreate" the current practice, as is. The proponents of this methodology contend that if a hospital was going to purchase a medical practice, then it should be valued at the price that it would take for that hospital to start that exact same medical practice. This approach always benefits the seller (the practice, in this case) because there is substantial investment to starting a medical practice: paying recruiting fees, initializing lines of credit to cover the periods of no-cash flow, providing income guarantees, and more.

A key theory behind this methodology of valuing goodwill is that when not dealing with an *efficient market,* as defined in the efficient market hypothesis, in which perfect information is available to all participants and an equal playing field exists between buyers and sellers with adequate liquidity, one must ultimately create an efficient market environment via a potentially complex model based on various assumptions and calculations. However, when applying this methodology, one must ask whether this model represents a true fair market value profile of the particular entity. Meaning, does that method yield a value that accurately reflects the amount that would result from the exchange of property between a willing buyer and willing seller?[1] In many cases, this method can yield very accurate results. Conversely, even the most complex and analytical-based quantitative models cannot accurately reflect the true dynamics of a fluid and evolving marketplace, particularly one involving assets with relatively little liquidity and/or marketability. This methodology cannot always adequately consider the true future value (ie, what may happen in the future as compared to what happened in the past).

Moreover, all of these calculations and models ultimately are based on assumptions derived by the valuator, and while some of the assumptions can be based on adequate standards and benchmarks, any model using this methodology will be highly subjective at best. As such, even though this methodology was heavily relied upon in the past, its applicability has since been outdated and, in most cases, will not provide an appraiser with a clear determinant of fair market value of an ongoing entity.

Research Through the Internet

The Internet has become a vital tool in improving the dissemination of information. In the appraisal industry, *accurate* information is king. Information available through the Internet is at a valuator's fingertips and is virtually unlimited. Any number of databases, studies, and other critical information can all be found there. The Internet has, in fact, proven to be an invaluable tool in the appraisal process.

In the days before the Internet, the research that was required to complete a valuation would take multiple hours of library, telephone, and interview work to ensure that nothing was missed. Now, information can readily be transferred from point to point, and reams of data that once were too costly to even maintain can now be stored in electronic format and downloaded by even the most computer-illiterate person. Software programs such as Adobe Acrobat®, Microsoft Word®, Microsoft Excel®, and myriad others have made the collection, storage, exchange, and (most importantly) the ability to understand and interpret information easier than ever before.

In addition to making information more available, the Internet has also made information and data more current. In the past, companies that published key market data would usually do so in large-volume books that were sold on an annual basis. This information usually had a one-year lag time (eg, if the book were published in one year, it was generally based on data from the previous year). Certainly this information is useful—at the time, it was the only way of providing it—but year-old data do not represent the timeliest information. The Internet, however, has largely eliminated the need for this time lag. Information can be updated on a regular basis as needed or as events occur. The need for a year's delay is gone, and information can (and should) be updated almost on a real-time basis.

An entire cottage industry has formed that focuses on providing real time, accurate market data to persons working within the financial markets and financial services firms. Many traditional media companies, such as Standard & Poor, McGraw Hill, Reuters, Bloomberg LP, The Economist Group, *Financial Times*, Dow Jones, *Wall Street Journal,* and Forbes have practically sustained their seemingly dying business model by providing financial data on a variety of companies. Furthermore, start-up companies focus on leveraging technology and using the Internet to provide database and analytics to market employees; these include Capital IQ, Dun & Bradstreet, Hoovers, Merger Market, and hundreds of others. Finally, the market research and analysis subsector, as a whole, has evolved to providing its services via the Internet and leveraging technology to enhance the quality and extensiveness of its products. Some firms that provide health care industry specific data include Levin Associates, Sullivan Cotter, and many investment banks that have research divisions with health care industry focus. Furthermore, many health care trade associations have invested heavily in collecting and aggregating data that can be applied to analysis for their members, including the Medical Group Management Association (MGMA), the American Medical Association, and the American Hospital Association, among other groups, including specialty associations.

The ease of application on the Internet is two-fold. Not only does it make information more available, but it also allows anyone with a computer, a telephone, and an opinion to become a self-appointed "expert." With such a simple medium (ie, the Internet) in which to work, virtually anyone can post information. Thus, the appraiser must take responsibility to gain an understanding of what is reasonable and realistic versus that which is meaningless.

For example, while someone may have performed a study of initial public offerings (IPO) that concluded a 110% premium for control ownership, this does not necessarily mean that it is an accurate study or that the results can be applied to any situation. For instance, what if the study was performed by Bob's Valuation and Pest Control? And what if Bob's study considered just two stocks over a period of 25 years? This study may not be the best one to reference when applying the rationale for a control premium.

Just because an article or study is posted on the Internet does not mean that it has any validity or that it bears any shred of truth. Most credible information is cited in a number of different places. For example, if an obscure review about a study performed 30 years prior was cited in passing and no mention of that review can be found elsewhere, the data and conclusions from such a study are likely not appropriate for application to a unique situation today. Likewise, if, while doing research on an issue, a specific study is constantly cited, chances are that that study is valid. Regardless, one should always verify information.

Another unfortunate outcome of Internet research is the amount of useless information that is provided. For every page of useful information found on the Internet, 20 pages will probably be useless. Whether it is supporting documentation or useless information, the researcher must be able to sift through it all and determine what is necessary and what is not. Internet research should be done quickly and proficiently, so that fees are not in question (see the appraisal fee section of Chapter 11). If the majority of the researcher's time is spent sorting through information rather than truly applying it, then the time spent on the project will exceed budget.

While we have outlined some of the obvious and concerning negative aspects of Internet-based research and data collection within the valuation process, this does not mean that a valuator should disregard online information. If credible, this information can be extremely advantageous and indeed accurate for a valuator. For instance, one of the benefits of using reputable online databases, such as Capital IQ and Bloomberg LP, is that the data are often verified and cited, and the user can typically distinguish between a data-point that was self-reported by a company versus information that was reported by a reputable news source or even directly from a stock exchange.

Another valuable aspect of using online resources is that many of the more advanced databases have custom-built software and cloud-based tools that allow the user to create custom quantitative models directly within that system. For instance, if the user sources economic and demographic data from the US Department of Labor's Bureau of Labor and Statistics, not only can models be constructed that extract specific metrics and data-points being sought, but they also can be downloaded directly into Microsoft® Excel and/or other analysis software, such as produced by SAS®.

Another example is the MGMA's annual Physician Production and Compensation Survey Report. The data from this survey, which has been widely adopted as one of the most reliable sources for medical practice benchmarks, are published in a voluminous printed version; however, they are also available via a proprietary software package that allows users to build custom models based on the specific data they are seeking. In the MGMA software, a setup assistant guides users through the process to produce a custom analysis that will generate various charts, graphs, and scatter plots to illustrate their results.

While these tools are very useful and advantageous because of their relative availability, one must still use caution when attempting to derive any sort of conclusions that are quantitatively or even scientifically sound. Not every analyst has to be the utmost quantitative expert or doctorate-level economist. However, the best and most valuable analysts and valuators are those who can incorporate a large volume of the most accurate quantitative data and combine it with the relevant qualitative variables to yield assumptions that have the least amount of volatility when changes are entered into the particular scenario. The rest is essentially mathematics. In essence, all valuators need to have a little bit of an economist, accountant, mathematician, statistician, and computer programmer in them. However, none of those traits is useful without the critical knowledge of the types of entities an appraiser is valuing and the dynamics of the markets in which those businesses operate.

The models themselves are essentially mathematical calculations that are incredibly simple when applied in a vacuum, which is why many people run into problems when attempting to value their own entities. It is easy to apply inputs to a model that provides an output result; however, if that model is not built on both reliable source data and appropriate assumptions, the results are meaningless.

The key to avoiding some of the pitfalls of using the Internet in valuation analysis is relatively straightforward; valuators should always verify any source of information and apply their own critical thinking process to any analysis to ensure that the context of that particular analysis is applicable to the current valuation subject. This principle can be applied to any aspect of research within the valuation process, including sources not limited to the Internet. Analysts should always consider the context of the information they are using, as well as the source, whether it is an online article, database, book published by a trade association found in the local library, or a direct interview discussion with an individual.

Operations Assessment

To perform a full valuation of an entity, especially in the health care industry, appraisers must have a detailed knowledge of that entity's operations. The operations have a direct influence on the entity's future earnings and how they will be affected in the future. The operational review and its depth will be commensurate with the size of the entity. For example, a smaller medical practice can be reviewed relatively quickly. However, a large hospital or nursing home may take considerably more time to review.

Furthermore, larger entities will inevitably require different skill sets and knowledge bases on the part of the appraisers, so a valuation team is often needed to value larger entities, rather than the one-person approach for smaller organizations. For instance, larger entities (ie, \$20 million or more in revenue) should only hire valuation firms that have specialists who focus on one or two specific valuation methodologies or approaches. Most health care facilities are asset-rich, meaning a significant amount of tangible assets are commonly involved with many facilities, such as hospitals, health systems, and long-term facilities. As such, it is likely a good idea to have someone who specializes in tangible asset valuations as part of the valuation team. Some valuations of tangible assets call for a highly specialized appraiser, called a machinery and engineering appraiser; these appraisers are often required to obtain a final valuation of assets on hospital transactions. Asset valuations involve conducting a detailed inventory of every tangible asset that an entity owns and can be extremely time-consuming; therefore, it is critical to have experts executing these processes. When adding unique types of equipment, such as magnetic resonance imaging, computed tomography, nuclear imaging, electrocardiography, and others, the specific experience valuing health care assets becomes critical for an entity to obtain an accurate valuation.

Another reason to procure an appraiser with thorough knowledge in health care is because operations play a large part in determining future earnings. Knowledge and understanding about how health care entities work, which can be quite different from the operations of other service entities, can provide a level of insight that a regular appraiser may not have.

Operations are key to understanding the subject company, and the assessment is essentially a broad overview of the entity's operations, and how those operations impact the financial and economic variables associated with that entity. When the appraiser is qualified to provide such services is often an ideal time for the entity to conduct a detailed operational study. Operations should be reviewed on a regular basis, conducted at the minimum of every five years, to ensure that operations are maintaining the highest levels of optimal efficiency. Some larger companies may even have their own internal auditing team that periodically reviews both financial and operational issues. Unfortunately, it is likely that smaller organizations cannot afford to allocate their own people, much less have a dedicated team, to review the organization's operations. Moreover, when an organization allocates internal personnel to the task, the reviewer may not have the knowledge to understand the broad range of issues or may be more reluctant to report mismanagement to the employer.

A detailed outside review can avert many of these issues. In addition, if an appraisal is being completed (either mutually or separately) by one organization that is looking to invest in or purchase all or a portion of another entity, the potential buyer should have the utmost concern for how that organization operates. This review process, called transaction due diligence, is one of the most critical elements of any transaction and the final value ascribed to it.

For example, if an orthopedic practice is considering the purchase of another practice, the orthopedic practice should be knowledgeable about the financial operations, billing and collections, personnel staffing and benefits, and the like, of the target entity. This is true with all service companies, but it is especially true within the health care industry, because the services and the operations that contribute to the production of those services are the underlying foundation of the entire business, and thus its value. These issues transcend a normal appraisal and move into what is commonly referred to as a detailed operational review.

A detailed operational review may consist of (but is not limited to) a review of any one of the following issues:

- Personnel review
- Revenue cycle analysis
- Internal controls and procedures
- Management information systems review
- Patient management analysis
- Regulatory and compliance analysis
- Facility review
- Demographic analysis

All of these issues are in addition to the detailed financial review that is completed to perform an appraisal; all of the variables derived throughout this process are ultimately incorporated into the analysis that drives all of the assumptions and variables within a valuation model. In fact, some companies will have an appraisal completed on a regular basis to evaluate the financial stability of the organization. This is an ideal time to perform a detailed operational review.

Valuation Data Checklist

Regardless of whether a detailed operations assessment will be completed, the appraiser requires a staggering amount of information to complete the valuation. Again, this exact information and the detail that is sought will be based on the extent of the valuation and the size of the entity. This information will vary based on the size of the entity and the scope of the review.

Conclusion

This chapter covers general items that are essential to the valuation process but not in the same categories with the previous topics of review. *Multiples*, *ratios*, *rules of thumb*, and *valuation methodologies* are more than merely jargon used by the competent appraiser. These terms are essential components of the project. This chapter also provides some useful information about resources available for gaining the necessary background to attain the needed ratios, multiples, and rules of thumb. This is the practical chapter that helps the appraiser complete the job for the client and helps the client accept the steps that are being taken with a measure of understanding.

Endnote

1. Internal Revenue Service. Revenue Ruling 59–60. Available at http://www.hantzmonwiebel.com/live_data/documents/ruling-59-60.pdf. Accessed June 10, 2011.

CHAPTER 11

Managing the Appraiser-Client Relationship

OUTLINE

- I. Introduction
- II. Managing the Appraiser
  - A. Know the Appraiser
    - 1. Finding a Qualified Appraiser
    - 2. Researching an Appraiser
  - B. Appraisal Fees
- III. Managing the Client
  - A. Fair and Independent
  - B. Knowledge Is Power
  - C. Expert Witness
- IV. Conclusion

Chapters 7 and 8 discuss each component of the valuation and valuation process. The process includes engaging an appraiser to calculate the values and considering the various standards and approaches that are available to complete the process. When a physician practice is sold and/or physicians are contracted to provide services with another hospital or health system, federal law dictates that the transaction and/or contractual arrangement be at a fair market value (FMV). The FMV requirements include the outright purchase and/or sale of an entity (as well as any type of lease, such as real estate rentals), leasing of assets, and hiring of staff. Other aspects of physicians' compensation with a hospital or health system must also be at FMV rates, including base salary, pay-for-call, medical directorships, and service-line management.

The appraiser is subject to and liable for Stark, federal anti-kickback, statute, and Internal Revenue Service (IRS) sanctions. If the approach used by an appraiser is in violation of legal guidelines, the appraiser could be subject to fines, penalties, exclusion from federal reimbursement programs, or other legal censure. In all of the prior discussions about valuations and obtaining an FMV opinion (discussed in Chapter 8), however, is the interaction between the appraiser (also referred to as a valuator) and the client. It should be noted that the *client* in an appraisal situation can be the entity that is being valued. However, the client can also refer to another entity that is a part of a transaction. This entity, such as a hospital or health system, must obtain an FMV opinion to ensure that the transaction and the associated agreements in which they are considering entering meet all applicable regulatory and legal requirements that govern such matters.

In assessing the value of a business entity, few books address the interaction between the client and the appraiser. Nevertheless, this relationship is an integral part of the process. Most texts do not include it because relationships are subjective. In general, positive interaction between the client and the appraiser is learned on the job or conveyed to new appraisers from those who are more experienced. Positive interaction is just as integral to the assignment as calculating an accurate discount rate or incorporating realistic assumptions into a pro forma model.

This chapter reviews some of the key areas that go beyond the actual valuation process and trend into more of the relationship phase of the project.

Managing the Appraiser

Managing the appraisal process begins with basic knowledge of the appraiser and the associated fees. To work well with appraisers, it is helpful for both parties to have a clear and mutual understanding of the role that a client has engaged the appraiser to fulfill. The role of valuator can change, depending on the client and the specific situation in which they are working. For instance, in many cases, appraisers serve as *valuation advisors*, which means they are representing the client in a transaction. They are specifically assigned to assist them determine an appropriate valuation for their entire entity or some other contractual element of a deal with another party. In this process, valuators function as a third party, with an obligation to represent the particular client who has engaged them in a manner that is compliant with both the terms of their agreement and all applicable regulations and laws.

The appraisers' work should be guided by appropriate standards and best practices, while also remaining compliant with appropriate regulatory requirements. However, appraisers will also work to guide the client toward the most optimal end of the reasonable range with which they are working to gain the most advantageous deal for the client.

Conversely, in some situations, valuators may be mutually engaged by multiple parties to serve the sole role of a completely independent party. In this case, valuators should assume the role of representing the interests of both parties throughout the transaction process. Nevertheless, the appraisers' work always should be guided first by appropriate standards directing the valuation and FMV process, with secondary consideration on how the client can benefit strategically or qualitatively. As such, the entities involved in a transaction should keep this in mind as they are working with appraisers, regardless of who engaged the work or who is paying the fee. Further, the entity that is engaging the appraiser should keep these principles in mind as they are writing an engagement agreement. In addition, they should have their legal counsel review the agreement prior to executing it to ensure that the agreement is compliant with appropriate standards.

Know the Appraiser

A vast number of people offer appraisal services and represent themselves as business appraisers. The field includes those who specialize in everything from widgets to wing nuts, and each field has its own methodologies and approaches that are more accepted than others. As discussed in Chapter 9, the income approach is identified as one of the most effective methods for valuing a medical practice. However, appraisers who specialize in real estate will probably never use a discounted cash flow (DCF) or the income approach because a business valuation and real estate valuation are two separate schools of value and use many varying techniques.

Anyone who has purchased a home has encountered an appraiser at some point; however, it is typically safe to assume that the individual who appraised your house is not the best person to render an opinion of FMV on a dynamic and complex business concern. Likewise, almost all of the largest financial services firms, investment banks, and public accounting firms have divisions that provide valuation and appraisal services. However, these services may not be appropriate for every situation, even if it involves a larger transaction, because those firms may not have individuals with adequate experience valuing similar or comparable entities within the health care industry.

Small firms will usually specialize in only one business field, whereas the larger firms will cover numerous fields and practices, as they are termed, within their appraisal department. Larger firms generally have an employee pool large enough to span the wide range of knowledge that is required in such an operation.

In general, when selecting an appraiser or valuation advisor, it is important to find someone who exhibits the skills and knowledge specific to the industry under consideration. Valuation firms are companies that specialize in doing business valuations in varying fields, whether it is a health care facility, such as a medical practice or hospital, or a multibillion dollar-a-year manufacturer of potato chips. The important point is not the size of the firm or really about the size of the entity being valued. Large or small, it is likely that the same processes and methodologies will be applied. What is critical is that the individual or team conducting a valuation be experienced and knowledgeable, specifically with a similar or comparable type of entity as the one under review in a specific transaction.

Finding a Qualified Appraiser

The first step should be to find a qualified and reputable valuation firm that knows the all aspects of health care facilities, including a medical practice, surgery center, or any other type of medical facility. Appraisers who know general business, or even those who specialize in services businesses, may not necessarily understand the business of health care services. For this reason, someone who is knowledgeable *both* in health care *and* appraising should be considered.

The field of medicine has its specialists and subspecialists (eg, a general surgeon and an orthopedic surgeon). Likewise, some appraisers also subspecialize. While some appraisers only value medical entities, some will have experience limited to one specialty (eg, surgery centers, radiology practices). This narrow focus may be acceptable, or it may be better to select appraisers with a broader base of experience. It might be a mistake to engage appraisers so focused on one field that they do not have a broad scope of what goes on in the rest of the medical industry. Typically, a qualified appraisal firm in the health care field will have adequate knowledge of any specialty, as well as a broad range of entity types (ie, clinical practice vs ancillary facility vs acute care facility).

When considering hiring an appraiser, clients should seek the recommendation of professional organizations and specialty societies and associations. These organizations can typically provide a list of competent valuation firms, or they likely have featured representatives from reputable firms as speakers at conferences. Also consider references from legitimate valuation-specific sources, such as the American Society of Appraisers and Chartered Financial Analyst Institute. Moreover, clients might seek referrals from colleagues who have recently had an appraisal conducted.

Nevertheless, a referral does not ensure that the recommended firm or appraiser is best suited or most qualified, especially in the medical field. Likewise, one colleague's appraiser may not be appropriate or qualified for all types of practices. For example, an appraiser may have received a high rating from a practice because the medical practice was valued at 10 times earnings before interest, taxes, depreciation, and amortization (EBITDA) rather than because the appraiser was competent and qualified. It is always possible that the appraiser valued that practice at 10 times EBITDA because of incompetence.

Researching an Appraiser

Researching appraisers should begin with obtaining an idea of what key parameters the valuation process will entail and specifically what resources will be sought from an appraiser. For instance, is the goal solely to find an individual or firm to "okay" a valuation? Or is the search for dynamic advisory services around what the value of the entity should be, which will then guide the term sheet and negotiation process when talking to potential buyers? In many larger transactions involving publicly traded companies, parties to the deal will often engage one of the so-called Big Four public accounting and audit firms for the sole reason of having their name attached to a deal saying that the value was acceptable for shareholders. This behavior was precisely what led to the destruction of Arthur Andersen, which was signing off on audits of Enron, when the company's books were obviously full of illegal practices, and other firms on unethical business corruption. Therefore, the reputation of a financial firm is the first and most critical issue to consider, because the specifics of the evaluation they conduct is not so proprietary or unique that they are the only ones who can do it.

The key aspect for clients is that these firms have apparently performed enough appraisals so that their particular experience and perspective is considered more valuable than others. Even though most medical groups are most likely smaller than a publicly-traded company, this discussion has become extremely relevant within the health care industry, as the government more closely scrutinizes even small transactions involving medical groups and health systems. Clients will often need a reputable firm to sign-off on the deal before it can close, or they will need a firm to sign-off on the deal to facilitate its progress through the regulatory approval process. In most of these cases, entities do not need to bring in a Big Four firm to provide the valuation, although they often do need a firm that has a successful and extensive track record providing such services with comparable entities and within similar deals.

One should always keep in mind that recommendations from a colleague, firm, or association do not mean that the valuation firm or individual is competent or qualified to value a medical entity. Unqualified appraisers and firms outnumber qualified ones; therefore, when hiring a firm to do an appraisal, clients should research possible candidates. Questions to ask an appraiser or firm include the following:

- Does the firm have any professional certifications?
- How long has the firm been doing appraisals?
- On average, how many appraisals does the firm do each year, etc?
- What types of health care services and provider valuations has the appraiser conducted? What appraisal methodologies are generally employed?

- Can you provide an example valuation report or other type of comparable deliverable that will likely be included in the particular engagement?

It is appropriate to probe a little further to discover what the appraisal firm knows about appraisals in the medical field. Some such questions may include the following:

- How would a relative value unit (RVU)-based compensation system affect the value?
- How have the recent Health Insurance Portability and Accountability Act (HIPAA) laws affected medical valuations?
- How does coding affect the valuation calculations, etc? How could changes in the coding structure (ie, evolution of International Statistical Classification of Diseases and Related Health Problems, 10th edition [ICD-10]) impact their valuation?

Lack of experience with detailed clinical issues does not mean that the appraisal firm does not know anything about health care appraisals. More than likely, it means the firm does not know anything about the clinical side of health care (and there is a difference). Ultimately, an appraisal firm that knows about RVUs, HIPAA, and Current Procedural Terminology (CPT®) will likely be well versed in the health care field. Likewise, the practice's certified public accountant (CPA), although knowledgeable in the fields of finance and accounting, may not be a skilled business appraiser, and in particular, may not be a qualified appraiser of a medical entity. A referral of an appraisal professional, whether from a client, firm, or association, should not be accompanied by a referral fee. Whether a firm provided competent appraisal services can often be swayed by a referral fee.

Appraisal Fees

Most appraisers will set hourly fees within the proposal for services or an engagement agreement (often referred to as the *engagement letter*). The full valuation typically is quoted, and hourly rates are held to the quoted maximum price, regardless of extra hours that may be incurred. Depending on the specific services involved in the engagement of a valuation advisor, the fees can have different structures, including an hourly or daily fee-for-service structure, total project fixed fee, or a straight *time and materials* structure that is based on a defined hourly rate, as mentioned.

All sizes of companies, whether large or small, need appraisers, and the appraiser fees should be priced accordingly. First, it must be understood that for a full, in-depth appraisal to be completed, a significant amount of due diligence has to be done. The completion of an appraisal is not simply the entering of a few numbers into a spreadsheet model that generates some magic number. As discussed in previous chapters, valuations are a combination of science and art. Most importantly, they involve a process that is dynamic and tailored to each individual situation with the application of consistent standards and practices applied to that process to ensure consistency and compliance with appropriate standards. If the appraisal is to be properly conducted, the client should be willing to make the investment in a competent appraiser because it almost undoubtedly will be beneficial to them in the end.

Managing the Client

The magnitude of work that goes into an appraisal for a smaller medical practice is typically not as substantial as that for a larger practice or hospital. However, since each process is unique, the valuator must be able to value objectively an entity by applying standard practices, regardless of size, scope, or scale. Nevertheless, simply due to the sheer size and magnitude of data involved in valuing larger entities, finalizing a valuation and/or FMV opinion for a large medical group or hospital will often require a larger valuation team. Furthermore, if an appraiser who specializes in the health care field is chosen, the appraisal process can proceed with greater ease, as that person is more knowledgeable in the field and is much better equipped to handle the research end of the appraisal.

If an appraisal is to be properly conducted, be ready to make the necessary investment. Beware of the appraiser who promises a detailed appraisal in 5 to 10 hours or who only needs to review a copy of the company's financials to provide "a number" for a full appraisal. Granted, if the practice only requires that calculations be made, then perhaps supplying financials is all that is warranted. Caution is advised. The level of the practice's involvement will be commensurate with the requirements of the project being completed.

No set amount of hours can be given as a benchmark, as they will change with every entity. As long as the proper due diligence is outlined in the proposal and completed and all of the approaches are considered, the client should reasonably be able to determine if the hours that are estimated are appropriate for the size of the entity.

Much like the appraiser who agrees to complete an appraisal in a very short period of time, the appraiser who seems to "move in" and never leave should also be avoided. Many larger practices pay exorbitant fees for professional service and knowledge. However, charging high fees and assigning a small army of consultants to the project do not ensure that a large firm will be any more effective than a smaller appraisal firm.

Fair and Independent

The appraiser must be aware that many times owners of a medical practice, especially a small medical practice, have dedicated their life to the practice. In such cases, appraisers must not allow the client to influence any decisions or outcomes.

Consider an appraisal being completed on a physician's majority ownership of a thriving surgery center for legal purposes (eg, divorce). While this physician may be honest and have integrity, at the same time, he or she may try to influence the final value of that ownership. Appraisers have to rise above any kind of undue influence and resist the client who tries to compromise the appraiser's professionalism. This situation is especially true in today's business environment, where business ethics commonly take on increasing importance.

The appraisal community, especially the medical appraisal community, is small, and bad news travels fast. If a consultant or firm is proven to be less than trustworthy in any of their dealings, legal actions may occur if any damage is committed, with reputational consequences. Appraisers should remain fair and independent and without reproach. The consultant/firm's reputation and ability to attract future clients relies on unwavering honesty and integrity.

Although it is unfortunate, clients are not going to be happy all of the time with the appraisers' report. This is especially true for medical practice appraisals, and even truer if the practice is small. Physicians often dedicate their lives to their practice, and when it comes time to appraise the value of that practice, the appraiser is the person relaying the bad news if the value falls short of expectations. Even if the practice had a considerable amount of value based on the appraisal (eg, $200,000), but the owners were under the impression that the medical practice should be selling closer to 10 times revenue (eg, closer to $1 million), the appraiser's value may cause some serious disagreements between the client and the appraiser.

If appraisers follow the rules and standards set forth, there may be some subjectivity that allows for disagreement (eg, the calculation of the discount rate under the income approach, the application of discounts and premiums), but with the proper due diligence and reasonable assumption outcomes, subjective decisions should be more than defendable.

If a legitimate error led to a mistake (eg, a considerable one-time expense that went unnoticed), the appraiser's fair and independent nature should not be impugned because of the oversight. It is difficult for an appraiser to learn everything about any entity, its history, and what comprises its operations with only a few days on-site, so it is likely that some misinterpretations may occur; if they do, the appropriate adjustments should be made.

Knowledge Is Power

Appraisers should provide detailed knowledge and understanding of all appraisal issues. They should be well adept in accounting, finance, and the industry in which the subject company operates. There are not many universities that offer degree programs specifically in business appraisal, although some schools have similar types of programs. Further, continuing education courses and certification programs are critical for appraisers. However, even with numerous educational opportunities available to a valuator of health care entities, much of the information that is learned is derived from on-the-job training and performing appraisals for actual clients.

Continuing education is a very important element in building a valuator's ongoing knowledge base and skill sets. In addition to post-graduate education, it also includes accreditation programs that specialize in business appraisal. In fact, these other accreditation programs are some of the most useful areas in which to receive continued education. Additional accreditation may be received from organizations such as the following:

- American Society of Appraisers (ASA)
- Chartered Financial Analysts Institute
- Institute of Business Appraisers
- American Institute of Certified Public Accountants
- Canadian Institute of Chartered Business Appraisers
- National Association of Certified Valuation Analysts

Any person who is choosing to go into the business appraisal field should strongly consider seeking accreditation with one of these associations.

Most people do not attend accreditation classes immediately after completing college. Instead, people will often spend a few years gaining experience before they make their career choice and choose the appraisal field. Thus, it may occur that someone who has not started the accreditation process is performing appraisals, which is fine as long as they are supervised by someone with the knowledge and understanding of the issues. There are many mundane financial analyses and research that must be completed in an appraisal process, and as long as the appraiser is competent and understands the process, there is no reason for concern. In fact, many of the larger firms conduct business in this manner.

Regardless of who is completing the work, the person who is responsible for and signs off on the report (see Chapter 2) should have a detailed knowledge and understanding of the appraisal process and know how the report was completed. Rarely will both parties interested in the outcome of the appraisal (ie, the seller and the buyer) be completely happy with the proposed number. Most of the time the seller will think the price is inordinately low, while the buyer will think it much too high. This is human dynamics.

When an appraisal is completed, appraisers have to be able to answer with certainty, clarity, and knowledge all questions about how the value was calculated. If they cannot, this inability may cast doubt on the appraiser and the legitimacy of the report.

It is imperative that the appraiser be skilled and knowledgeable in all areas of business appraisal. For example, if, during a presentation meeting, the appraiser is asked why a certain methodology under the asset-based approach was not applied, the answer to this question must be thoughtfully and concisely forthcoming. If there is a question as to why a premium or discount was applied via a market valuation, the appraiser should be able to answer that question, citing one of the many supporting studies to bolster the reply.

Again, subjectivity enters into every report, but if the appraiser can cite evidence and supporting documentation as to why or why not an approach was applied, the final calculation will be all the more refutable.

Expert Witness

In the event a lawsuit is filed, appraisers may be called as expert witnesses. First and foremost, it must be said that not everyone is appropriate to serve as an expert witness. Attorneys and appraisers are often teamed together or against one another to defend an appraisal. Although work as an expert witness is challenging, it can often be very daunting when it appears that an attorney's sole purpose is to prove a case against the appraiser.

As noted, often the two parties in an appraisal will disagree as to the value of the entity in question. In a normal appraisal case, this situation may occur; but in expert witness work, it is almost always true. Whether the attorney is trying to discredit the appraisal or another appraiser has been hired by the other side to testify, the validity of the appraisal is in question.

In this case, the other side (ie, the attorney or appraiser) is going to look for the smallest detail that may have been missed, as a means to have the original opinion taken out of consideration. When or if that detail is found, it could be challenging to defend the project. Even that smallest detail can be enough to defeat the entire appraisal. The best rule of thumb for appraisers choosing to appear as an expert witness is to go into a project thoroughly prepared. When working as an expert witness in the appraisal field, appraisers must be intimately knowledgeable with regard to *all* issues of business appraisal, including the ability to cite resources, back up and verify all information, and pinpoint every method's applicability in the business appraisal. Appraisers should not only be informed of business appraisal standards but also of relevant legal and regulatory requirements that might impact their methods, practices, and conclusions. If the appraisal's methods include some level of subjectivity, the appraiser can tell the opposing attorney that even the courts recognize that "valuation is necessarily an approximation and a matter of judgment, rather than of mathematics."[1]

Conclusion

Whether client or appraiser, both roles have duties and responsibilities to fulfill. Clients have the obligation to choose the appropriate appraiser and do the sufficient research to make sure that the person or firm they choose is competent and understands business appraisal.

Clients should focus on a firm or individual who will provide the services that are needed within a reasonable fee structure. Most firms will provide fees on an at-risk basis, but it is the client's role to understand the value of investing in a competent appraiser. Do not expect to get a full, adequately prepared document for just a few thousand dollars. There is a required level of due diligence that appraisers have to perform, and if someone promises to complete the work for a lower price, then it is likely that the finished product will be of lesser quality.

Clients must be honest with the appraiser. Although every appraiser would like the final product to be joyfully accepted, no appraiser should tolerate undue influence from the client. Likewise, clients should not change the deliverable half way through a project and then expect the appraiser to not adjust the cost accordingly.

As clients have obligations, so too do appraisers. If a deliverable is promised, the appraiser is obligated to provide it within the agreed upon timeframe. If the appraiser has priced the project too low, no corners should be cut to complete the final report. Appraisers have ethical and legal obligations that cannot be avoided or minimized.

Professionals who choose to pursue a career in the appraisal business should learn every aspect of the business. Receiving the proper accreditations should be a goal; some have argued that accreditations should even be mandatory for people to provide appraisal services, similar to that of an accountant or lawyer. Maintaining knowledge on changes within the industry and continuing education should always be priorities. In many cases, potential clients seeking the counsel of a competent valuation advisor will set the bar of qualifications where they feel it is most appropriate. Therefore, even if certain degrees and/or certifications are not technically required to perform these services, the majority of health care executives today will only work with firms and individuals who bring diversified skills, credentials, and overall value to the table.

Endnote

1. *Davis v Commissioner*, 110 TC 530,554 (1998). Citing from *Hamm v Commissioner*, 325 F2d 940.

CHAPTER 12 Regulations in the Appraisal of Health Care Enterprises

OUTLINE

I. Introduction
II. Tax Exempt Organization Issues
  A. Organizations Exempt from Taxation
  B. Restriction Against Private Inurement
  C. Public Benefit
III. Federal Anti-Kickback Statute
  A. Criminal Prohibition
  B. Safe Harbors
IV. Stark Law
  A. Fair Market Value
  B. Commercial Reasonableness
  C. Exceptions
V. Conclusion

Inasmuch as health care is among the most heavily regulated industries in the country, a number of federal regulations are applicable to the valuation of health care enterprises. Such regulations generally include among their provisions a requirement that health care-related transactions be executed at fair market value (FMV). Failure to satisfy the FMV requirement may result in significant liability to one or more of the parties to the transaction. This chapter provides a brief overview of

---

Disclaimer: The information in this chapter is not intended to be legal or tax advice. For legal or tax advice, readers should consult an attorney.

some of the more significant regulations that must be considered in relation to the valuation of health care enterprises.

Tax Exempt Organization Issues

Hospitals and other health care providers organized and operated exclusively for charitable purposes that are qualified for tax exempt status pursuant to section 501(c)(3) of the Internal Revenue Code (IRC) are subject to Internal Revenue Service (IRS) rules and regulations governing the activities and transactions of such providers. This section includes a general overview of some important issues applicable to tax exempt organizations in connection with arrangements involving such organizations and related valuations.

Organizations Exempt from Taxation

An organization described in IRC section 501(c)(3) may be exempt from taxation.[1] In the case of a hospital or other health care provider, in order to qualify for tax exempt status, that organization must be organized and operated exclusively for charitable purposes and no part of its net earnings shall inure to the benefit of any private shareholder or individual.[2] This requirement includes both an organizational component and an operational component. Treasury regulation section 1.501(c)(3) sets forth the requirements necessary to satisfy both the organizational and operational tests.[3]

In addition to the several organizational requirements set forth in the regulation, part of the organizational test addresses the distribution of organizational assets on dissolution.[4] "An organization is not organized exclusively for one or more exempt purposes unless its assets are dedicated to an exempt purpose."[5] The regulation requires that on dissolution of the organization, either pursuant to the organization's governing documents or by operation of law, the assets of the organization be distributed in a manner that would accomplish the general purposes for which the organization was formed. "An organization does not meet the organizational test if its articles or the law of the State in which it was created provide that its assets would, upon dissolution, be distributed to its members or shareholders."[6]

Under the operational test of the regulation,[7] the organization is required to engage primarily in activities that accomplish one or more exempt purposes, as specified in section 501(c)(3).[8] An organization will fail this test if more than "an insubstantial part of its activities is not in furtherance of an exempt purpose."[9] With respect to the distribution of earnings, the operational test is not met if any part of the net earnings inure to the benefit of private shareholders or individuals.[10]

In general, the tax exempt organization must serve a public rather than a private interest. To meet the regulatory requirement, therefore, the organization must establish "that it is not organized or operated for the benefit of private interests such as designated individuals, the creator or his family, shareholders of the organization, or persons controlled, directly or indirectly, by such private interests."[11]

Restriction Against Private Inurement

To have tax exempt status, no part of an organization's net earnings shall inure to the benefit of any private shareholder or individual. The term *private shareholders or individuals* is defined as persons having a personal and private interest in the activities of the organization.[12] This restriction against private inurement is generally applicable, therefore, to insiders with a relationship to the organization that allows some degree of control or influence over its activities.

The prohibition against inurement may apply to physicians who are determined to be insiders, that is, in a position to exercise control with respect to the exempt organization. In the context of the sale of a medical practice, any amount received by such a physician that is above the FMV of the practice's assets could be considered to have inured to the benefit of the physician. Such inurement may cause the organization to be ineligible for tax exempt status. Even if physicians are not considered to be insiders due to the absence of control, their receipt of excessive private benefits could cause the organization to be operated for private benefit rather than public benefit.[13]

Public Benefit

The requirement that a tax exempt organization, organized and operated exclusively for charitable purposes, serve a public benefit rather than a private benefit must be considered in transactions in which physicians sell their practice's assets to a tax exempt organization and subsequently perform services for such organization.[14] The concept of private benefit is broader than private inurement. While inurement generally involves a benefit from a tax exempt organization being received by an insider, a private benefit may not involve an insider but may involve a benefit to any party. In the case of the sale of a medical practice involving a tax exempt organization, therefore, the parties to the transaction will need to make sure that the valuation is properly performed and well documented to help prevent the conferring of an improper private benefit.[15]

The valuation of a practice's assets is very important, therefore, in determining whether private inurement or private benefit has occurred that could jeopardize the tax exempt status of an organization or trigger IRS sanctions on improper transactions and certain persons with respect to such transactions and organization.[16] As discussed in previous chapters, therefore, determining the FMV of assets and services in health care transactions is extremely important. The IRS definition of FMV, as set forth in Revenue Ruling 59-60 (RR 59-60), has been discussed in previous chapters. A more detailed discussion of the issues involving tax exempt organizations and applicable rules and regulations is beyond the scope of this book. All parties to transactions or arrangements involving tax exempt organizations should consult qualified legal and tax counsel for advice. The following sections of this chapter will discuss some additional regulations as they relate to the valuation of health care assets.

Federal Anti-Kickback Statute

The federal anti-kickback statute provides in part that:

> (1) "Whoever knowingly and willingly solicits or receives any remuneration (including any kickback, bribe, or rebate) directly or indirectly, overtly or covertly, in cash or in kind-
>
> (A) in return for referring an individual to a person for the furnishing or arranging for the furnishing of any item or service for which payment may be made in whole or in part under a Federal health care program, or
>
> (B) in return for purchasing, leasing, ordering, or arranging for or recommending purchasing, leasing, or ordering any good, facility, service, or item for which payment may be made in whole or in part under a Federal health care program,
>
> shall be guilty of a felony and upon conviction thereof, shall be fined not more than $25,000 or imprisoned for not more than five years, or both.
>
> (2) Whoever knowingly and willingly offers or pays any remuneration (including any kickback, bribe, or rebate) directly or indirectly, overtly or covertly, in cash or in kind to any person to induce such person-
>
> (A) to refer an individual to a person for the furnishing or arranging for the furnishing of any item or service for which payment may be made in whole or in part under a Federal health care program, or
>
> (B) to purchase, lease, order, or arrange for or recommend purchasing, leasing, or ordering any good, facility, service, or item for which payment may be made in whole or in part under a Federal health care program,
>
> shall be guilty of a felony and upon conviction thereof, shall be fined not more than $25,000 or imprisoned for not more than five years, or both."[17]

The Office of Inspector General (OIG) of the US Department of Health and Human Services is responsible for enforcing the anti-kickback statute.

Criminal Prohibition

The anti-kickback statute is a criminal prohibition against payments in any form that are intended to induce or reward referrals for services under Medicare, Medicaid, or any other federal health care program.[18] The statute is broad in scope and covers both the offer and payment of anything of value, as well as the solicitation and receipt of anything of value for referrals or other generation of business payable in whole or in part by a federal health care program.[19] In addition to criminal liability under the statute, violators also may be subject to civil money penalties and exclusion from participation in federal health care programs. Violation of the anti-kickback statute also may trigger liability under the False Claims Act[20] in situations in which the violation results in a claim for payment being submitted pursuant to a federal health care program.

Liability under the anti-kickback statute depends on the party's intent, that is, whether the party acted knowingly and willfully. The OIG Supplemental Compliance Program Guidance for Hospitals ("OIG Compliance Guidance"), while recognizing that liability under the anti-kickback statute is intent based, provides a two-step test for analyzing a practice or arrangement under the anti-kickback statute .[21] Under this analysis, a hospital would determine if any remunerative relationships exist between itself (or its affiliate or representatives) and persons or entities in a position to generate federal health care program business for the hospital (or its affiliates), directly or indirectly. Examples of such persons or entities include physicians, other health care professionals, ambulance companies, clinics, hospices, home health agencies, nursing facilities, and other hospitals.[22]

The next question is, with respect to any such relationships, "could *one purpose* of the remuneration be to induce or reward the referral or recommendation of business payable in whole or in part by a federal health care program?"[23] If so, the anti-kickback statute is implicated, and the arrangement must be carefully scrutinized by the hospital. The OIG Compliance Guidance provides additional questions that a hospital should ask about any arrangement or practice that has been identified as potentially problematic. Such analysis may be useful in assessing the risk of prosecution with respect to an arrangement or practice.[24]

According to the OIG Compliance Guidance, under the anti-kickback statute *one- purpose* test, neither a legitimate business purpose for the arrangement nor a fair market value payment will legitimize a payment if there also is an illegal purpose.[25] In the case of the acquisition by a hospital of the assets of a medical practice in which the payment is based on the FMV of such assets, if the hospital made the payment also for the purpose of inducing referrals payable under a federal health care program, thereby indicating the necessary intent, the anti-kickback statute has likely been violated.

The OIG also has recognized that generally "fair market value arrangements that are arm's-length and do not take into account in any manner the volume or value of federal health care program business, or arrangements that do not have as one purpose the generation of business payable by a federal health care program, should not raise concerns under the anti-kickback statute."[26] Again, the need to determine the FMV in such arrangements or transactions is critical.

In situations in which a hospital or its affiliate acquires a physician practice and the physicians in such practice continue to be affiliated with the hospital through employment or some other arrangement, the OIG has expressed significant concerns under the anti-kickback statute. The OIG has indicated the need to scrutinize the amounts paid for the practice or as compensation for services to determine whether they reasonably reflect the FMV of the practice or the services rendered. "To the extent that a payment exceeds the fair market value of the practice or the value of the services rendered, it can be inferred that the excess amount paid over fair market value is intended as payment for the referral of program-related business."[27] In determining what constitutes FMV of a physician practice, the OIG has indicated that any amount paid in excess of the FMV of "the hard assets of a physician practice would be open to question."[28] This further emphasizes the need for a thorough independent valuation of the practice and its assets to determine FMV. Any intangible value involved should be closely analyzed and documented as part of the independent valuation.

Safe Harbors

While the anti-kickback statute and the corresponding regulations provide for several safe harbors for common business arrangements, only one is directly applicable to certain sales of physician practices.[29] This safe harbor applies to certain sales made by a practitioner to another practitioner, and to a limited category of acquisitions of a practice by a hospital. The safe harbor does not apply to the acquisition of a practice by a hospital in which the practitioner continues to provide services to the hospital as an employee or otherwise, or in which the selling practitioner is otherwise in a professional position after the sale to make or influence referrals to, or otherwise generate business for, the purchasing hospital or entity for which payment may be made under a federal health care program.[30] The safe harbor for practitioner to practitioner sales provides the following:

> (e) Sale of practice
>
> (1) As used in section 1128B of the Act, "remuneration" does not include any payment made to a practitioner by another practitioner where the former practitioner is selling his or her practice to the later practitioner, as long as both of the following two standards are met-
>
> (i) The period from the date of the first agreement pertaining to the sale to the completion of the sale is not more than one year.

(ii) The practitioner who is selling his or her practice will not be in a professional position to make referrals to, or otherwise generate business for, the purchasing practitioner for which payment may be made in whole or in part under Medicare, Medicaid, or other Federal health care programs after 1 year from the date of the first agreement pertaining to the sale.[31]

In response to a proposed rulemaking, some commenters urged the OIG to expand the sale of practice safe harbor to protect sales of practices in accordance with FMV transactions and sales of practices to entities in connection with the creation of integrated health care delivery systems. OIG was further urged to modify the safe harbor to provide that reasonable valuation of all assets, tangible and intangible, may be used to determine the FMV of a practice.[32] In declining to modify the sale of practice safe harbor in such ways, the OIG indicated that while it did not intend to stand in the way of integrated delivery system acquisition of practices, concerns remained that "many such arrangements may provide incentives for overutilization, increased billings to the Federal programs, and inappropriate steering of patients."[33] The OIG also declined to provide safe harbor protection for any particular valuation methodology and stated its view that "payments for 'intangibles' can easily be used to disguise payments for referrals of Federal health care program business."[34]

The OIG has emphasized that safe harbor protection requires strict compliance with all applicable conditions contained in the safe harbor.[35] Compliance with a safe harbor is, however, voluntary. Failure to comply with a safe harbor does not necessarily mean that an arrangement is illegal. Any arrangement that does not fit within a safe harbor will need to be evaluated on a case-by-case basis.[36]

Stark Law

The federal physician self-referral law, also known as the Stark law,[37] prohibits a physician from referring patients for certain designated health services (DHS) that are payable under Medicare or Medicaid to an entity with which the physician or the physician's immediate family member has a financial relationship, including an ownership or compensation relationship, unless an exception under the law applies to the relationship. Any entity that provides such referred services is prohibited from filing a claim with Medicare or billing any individual, third-party payer, or other entity for the services.[38]

The purpose of the Stark law was to limit the impact of financial motivations on the part of physicians when referring patients for certain health services. Prior to the Stark law, studies had shown that physicians who had financial relationships with entities to which they referred ordered more services than those physicians without such financial relationships. It was the "correlation between financial ties and increased utilization" that prompted the Stark law.[39]

Under the Stark law, no wrongful intent or culpable conduct is required.[40] If the referral occurs and a financial relationship exists, then the Stark law is violated, unless the relationship fits within an exception. The law and its implementing regulations are complex, and because it is a strict liability law, even the smallest of technical violations can result in significant financial consequences.[41] Stark law violations also can result in civil penalties under the False Claims Act.

Fair Market Value

Unlike the anti-kickback statute, the Stark law provides a definition of FMV as follows:

> Fair market value means the value in arm's-length transactions, consistent with the general market value. "General market value" means the price that an asset would bring as the result of bona fide bargaining between well-informed buyers and sellers who are not otherwise in a position to generate business for the other party, or the compensation that would be included in a service agreement as the result of bona fide bargaining between well-informed parties to the agreement who are not otherwise in a position to generate business for the other party, on the date of acquisition of the asset or at the time of the service agreement. Usually, the fair market price is the price at which bona fide sales have been consummated for assets of like type, quality, and quantity in a particular market at the time of acquisition, or the compensation that has been included in bona fide service agreements with comparable terms at the time of the agreement, where the price or compensation has not been determined in any manner that takes into account the volume or value of anticipated or actual referrals. With respect to rentals and leases described in §411.357(a), (b), and (l) (as to equipment leases only), "fair market value" means the value of rental property for general commercial purposes (not taking into account its intended use). In the case of a lease of space, this value may not be adjusted to reflect the additional value the prospective lessee or lessor would attribute to the proximity or convenience to the lessor when the lessor is a potential source of patient referrals to the lessee. For purposes of this definition, a rental payment does not take into account intended use if it takes into account costs incurred by the lessor in developing or upgrading the property or maintaining the property or its improvements.[42]

In commenting on valuation methodologies and the definition of FMV, the Centers for Medicare and Medicaid Services (CMS), the federal agency responsible for enforcing the Stark law, has indicated that FMV is determined based on facts and circumstances. The appropriate valuation methodology depends on the nature of the transaction, its location, and other factors.[43] CMS has recognized that the Stark law covers a wide range of transactions and declined to comment definitively on any particular valuation methodology.[44] No particular valuation methodology, therefore, is mandated by the Stark law.

In subsequent rulemaking by CMS with respect to the Stark law, the agency noted its view that, in most cases, FMV for an item or service will be expressed as a range, and, therefore, claimants should not have significant difficulty in establishing FMV, provided that they use a methodology that is reasonable under the facts and circumstances, pay an amount that is within the range indicated by such methodology, and maintain documentation regarding the valuation that was created at the time of the transaction.[45]

In response to requests to clarify the documentation necessary to establish a transaction consistent with FMV, CMS indicated that it intended to accept any method that is commercially reasonable and provides evidence that the amount paid is comparable to the amount ordinarily paid for an item or service in the relevant location by parties operating at arm's-length who are not in a position to refer to one another.[46] It was indicated that the amount of documentation needed to confirm FMV will vary, depending on the circumstances in a given case and that there is no rule of thumb applicable in all situations.[47]

CMS was requested in a rulemaking process to confirm that internally generated surveys are sufficient to establish market value and that an independent valuation is not required. CMS indicated that although there is no requirement that parties engage an independent valuation consultant when other appropriate valuation methods are available, internally generated surveys are susceptible to manipulation and, absent independent verification, such surveys do not have strong evidentiary value and may be subject to more intensive scrutiny than an independent survey.[48] As previously emphasized, therefore, an independent third-party valuation is a critical step in the process of establishing FMV.

Commercial Reasonableness

In the preamble to a Stark law rulemaking, CMS defined the term "commercially reasonable" as it is used in the Stark law and its regulations as follows:

> An arrangement will be considered "commercially reasonable" in the absence of referrals if the arrangement would make commercial sense if entered into by a reasonable entity of similar type and size and a reasonable physician (or family member or group practice) of similar scope and specialty, even if there were no potential DHS referrals.[49]

Much like the determination of FMV, determining whether an arrangement is commercially reasonable requires a methodology that is reasonable under the relevant facts and circumstances and there is no single bright-line test. The requirement of commercial reasonableness is applicable to several of the exceptions contained in the Stark law.

Exceptions

As discussed, no wrongful intent or culpable conduct is required under the Stark law for a violation to occur. The Stark law is violated if the referral occurs and a financial relationship exists, unless the relationship fits within an exception. The Stark law and its regulations provide for several different types of exceptions. Some of the most significant exceptions in the context of the sale of a physician practice and the potential continuing relationship between the buyer and the seller include the exceptions for: (i) bona fide employment relationships, (ii) personal service arrangements, (iii) fair market value compensation, (iv) in-office ancillary services, and (v) academic medical centers.[50] This is not a complete list of all of the Stark law exceptions, or even those that may be applicable to the continuing relationship between a buyer and seller of a practice. All of the exceptions under the Stark law are contained in the Stark law regulations at 42 C.F.R. § 411.350 *et seq.*

Although we will not review the details of these exceptions, we will look briefly at the situation in which a hospital acquires a practice and then employs the selling physician. In this case, the post-acquisition employment relationship between the buyer and the seller would likely need to fit within the bona fide employment relationship exception to comply with the Stark law. The requirements of such exception are as follows:

> For purposes of § 411.353, the following compensation arrangements do not constitute a financial relationship:
>
> . . .
>
> (c) Bona fide employment relationships. Any amount paid by an employer to a physician (or immediate family member) who has a *bona fide* employment relationship with the employer for the provision of services if the following conditions are met:
>
> (1) The employment is for identifiable services.
>
> (2) The amount of the remuneration under the employment is –
>
> (i) Consistent with the fair market value of the services; and
>
> (ii) Except as provided in paragraph (c)(4) of this section, is not determined in a manner that takes into account (directly or indirectly) the volume or value of referrals by the referring physician.
>
> (3) The remuneration is provided under an agreement that would be commercially reasonable even if no referrals were made to the employer.[51]

As stated in the regulation, it will be necessary to determine both the FMV and the commercial reasonableness of the remuneration to determine if the relationship fits within the exception.

In the process of amending the Stark law exception for FMV compensation, and as part of the rulemaking process, CMS was requested to provide bright-line guidance as to what constitutes FMV and to establish a rebuttable presumption that a transaction is FMV. In declining to do so, CMS stated its view that the parties to a transaction or arrangement are in the best position to ensure that the remuneration is at FMV and to document such valuation at the time of the transaction or arrangement. CMS further stated that if questioned by the government, the burden would be on the parties to explain how the transaction or arrangement meets the FMV requirements.[52]

Conclusion

This chapter has provided a brief overview of some of the more significant regulations related to the valuation of health care enterprises. The regulations and issues discussed here are by no means all those that will need to be considered in the selling, closing, and valuation of a health care organization, or the valuation of a health care-related transaction or arrangement. For example, the other fraud and abuse laws, such as the False Claims Act and the Civil Money Penalty statute, must be considered. Other issues to be considered include, but are not limited to, those arising from or related to (i) the Patient Protection and Affordable Care Act (2010) and health care reform, including expansion of requirements applicable to hospitals for federal tax exempt status, accountable care organizations (ACOs), expansion of liability under fraud and abuse laws, and possible regulatory changes regarding the anti-kickback statute and Stark law, (ii) health information privacy and security laws and regulations, (iii) income tax laws, and (iv) state laws, such as those related to tax exempt status, anti-kickback, physician self-referral, and other prohibitions related to fraud and abuse. In all matters involving legal and tax considerations and issues, including those discussed in this chapter, it is critically important to consult a qualified attorney for specific legal advice.

The health care landscape is changing fast. At present, the health care industry is awaiting important finalized regulations and guidance to be issued by CMS and other federal agencies related to the creation of a Medicare shared savings program, the development of ACOs, and other health care reform initiatives. As the industry moves toward the greater integration envisioned by such initiatives, some of the regulations discussed in this chapter may be amended in response to the changing environment. As always, and especially in the midst of rapid changes, an independent third-party appraiser who is qualified and experienced in the analysis and valuation of health care organizations, assets, transactions, and arrangements, should be used to determine FMV and commercial reasonableness.

Endnotes

1. 26 USC § 501(a),(c)(3) (2009).
2. Ibid.
3. Treas Reg § 1.501(c)(3)-1 (2009).
4. Treas Reg § 1.501(c)(3)-1(b)(4) (2009).
5. Ibid.
6. Ibid.
7. Treas Reg § 1.501(c)(3)-1(c) (2009).
8. Treas Reg § 1.501(c)(3)-1(c)(1) (2009).
9. Ibid.
10. Treas Reg § 1.501(c)(3)-1(c)(2) (2009).
11. Treas Reg § 1.501(c)(3)-1(d)(1)(ii) (2009).
12. Treas Reg § 1.501(a)-1(c) (2009).
13. Gitterman JE, Friedlander M. *Health Care Provider Reference Guide.* IRS Exempt Organization Continuing Professional Education Text (2004 EO CPE Text). Available at www.irs.gov/pub/irs-tege/eotopicc04.pdf.
14. Treas Reg § 1.501(c)(3)-1(d)(1)(ii).
15. Gitterman JE and Friedlander M. *Health Care Provider Reference Guide.* IRS Exempt Organization Continuing Professional Education Text (2004 EO CPE Text). Available at www.irs.gov/pub/irs-tege/eotopicc04.pdf.
16. 26 USC § 4958 (2009).
17. 42 USC§ 1320a-7b(b)(1) and (2) (2009).
18. Office of Inspector General. Supplemental Compliance Program Guidance for Hospitals. *Fed Reg.* 2005; 70(No. 19):4858-76.
19. Ibid at 4864.
20. 42 USC § 1320a-7b(a) (2009); and 31 U.S.C.§ 3729 (2009) *et seq.*
21. Office of Inspector General. Supplemental Compliance Program Guidance for Hospitals. *Fed Reg.* 2005; 70(No. 19):4858-76.
22. Ibid.
23. Ibid.
24. Ibid.
25. Ibid.
26. Office of Inspector General. Medicare and State Health Care Programs: Fraud and Abuse; Safe Harbors for Certain Electronic Prescribing and Electronic Health Records Arrangements Under the Anti-Kickback Statute. *Fed Reg.* 2006; 71(No. 152):45110-11.
27. Thornton DM, Associate General Counsel, Inspector General Division. Response to Sullivan TJ, Technical Assistant (Health Care Industries), Office of the Associate Chief Counsel, Internal Revenue Service, regarding the views of the Office of Inspector General concerning the application of the federal anti-kickback statute to certain types of acquisitions of physi-

cian practices. Letter. December 22, 1992. *Available at* http://oig.hhs.gov/fraud/docs/safeharborregulations/acquisition122292.htm.

28. Ibid, 3.
29. 42 CFR § 1001.952(e) (2010).
30. Ibid.
31. 42 CFR § 1001.952(e)(1) (2010).
32. Office of Inspector General. Medicare and State Health Care Programs: Fraud and Abuse; Clarification of the Initial OIG Safe Harbor Provisions and Establishment of Additional Safe Harbor Provisions Under the Anti-Kickback Statute. *Fed Reg.* 1999; 64(No. 223):63518- 50.
33. Ibid, 63550.
34. Ibid. Emphasis in original.
35. Office of Inspector General. Supplemental Compliance Program Guidance for Hospitals. *Fed Reg.* 2005; 70(No. 19):4858-76.
36. Ibid.
37. 42 USC § 1395nn (2009).
38. 42 USC § 1395nn(a)(1) (2009).
39. Healthcare Financing Administration. Medicare and Medicaid Programs; Physicians' Referrals to Health Care Entities With Which They Have Financial Relationships. *Fed Reg.* 2001; 66 (No. 3):859–60.
40. Ibid.
41. *See* 42 USC § 1395nn (2009) *et seq,* and 42 CFR § 411.350 (2010) *et seq.*
42. 42 CFR § 411.351 (2010). Emphasis in original.
43. Centers for Medicare and Medicaid Services. Medicare Program; Physicians' Referrals to Health Care Entities With Which They Have Financial Relationships (Phase III). *Fed Reg.* 2007; 72(No. 171):51012, 51015-16
44. Ibid, 51016.
45. Centers for Medicare and Medicaid Services. Medicare Program; Changes to the Hospital Inpatient Prospective Payment Systems and Fiscal Year 2009 Rates; Payments for Graduate Medical Education in Certain Emergency Situations; Changes to Disclosure of Physician Ownership in Hospitals and Physician Self-Referral Rules; Updates to the Long-Term Care Prospective Payment System; Updates to Certain IPPS-Excluded Hospitals; and Collection of Information Regarding Financial Relationships Between Hospitals. *Fed Reg.* 2008; 73 (No. 154):48434, 48,739.
46. Healthcare Financing Administration. Medicare and Medicaid Programs; Physicians' Referrals to Health Care Entities With Which They Have Financial Relationships. *Fed Reg.* 2001; 66 (No. 3):856, 944
47. Ibid, 944.
48. Ibid, 945.
49. Centers for Medicare and Medicaid Services. Medicare Program; Physicians' Referrals to Health Care Entities With Which They Have Financial Relationships (Phase II). *Fed Reg.* 2004; 69(No. 59):16054, 16093.

50. 42 CFR § 411.355 (2010), and 42 CFR § 411.357 (2010).
51. 42 CFR § 411.357(c)(1)-(3) (2010).
52. Centers for Medicare and Medicaid Services. Medicare Program; Physicians' Referrals to Health Care Entities With Which They Have Financial Relationships (Phase III). *Fed Reg.* 2007; 72(No. 171):51012, 51060.

CHAPTER 13

Preparing the Practice for Maximum Value

OUTLINE

I. Introduction
II. Growth in Revenue and Productivity through Payment Strategies
    A. Evaluating the Payer Mix
        1. Enhancing the Payer Mix
        2. Developing a Balanced Payer Mix
    B. Fee Schedule Analysis
        1. Medicare
    C. Managed Care Implications
        1. Primary Care Practices
        2. Specialty Care Practices
    D. Productivity Standards
    E. Referral Patterns
    F. Compensation Incentives
    G. Provider Stability
III. Enhancing Value through Expense Controls
    A. Controlling Operating Expenses
        1. Salaries and Benefits
        2. Administrative Overhead
    B. Physician Compensation and Benefits
    C. Enhancing Value through Strategic Planning
    D. Personnel Policies and Procedures Manual
IV. Conclusion

It is becoming increasingly difficult for sole practitioners (or even medium-sized multispecialty groups) to survive and subsequently excel without consideration of partnering with other like-minded practice entities. Attaining peak value is the goal of an owner of any business. Medical practice ownership is no different, especially in preparation for such a transaction. Enacting sound business practices will ensure improved operating results and subsequently increase the marketability of the practice.

The purpose of this chapter is to offer practical guidance for optimizing the value of a medical practice in preparation for an acquisition. However, the following initiatives should be an ongoing part of the practice's business strategy, regardless of whether the owner intends to sell or just maintain market value. Maintaining a practice in excellent condition could be compared to maintaining real estate in maximum condition to capitalize on its value. Meanwhile, the owner enjoys optimum returns and benefits in the duration of ownership and is always prepared to sell as an opportunity arises.

Preparing the practice for maximum value involves several areas of management, including the following:

- Growth in revenue
- Productivity improvement
- Management and ultimate control of expenses
- Strategic planning and consideration of future initiatives

Growth in Revenue and Productivity through Payment Strategies

Obtaining fair and optimal payment from payers for a medical practice is a most important initiative for the long-term economic viability—if not survivability—of a practice. One way a practice can prepare to maximize its value is to establish an effective revenue base, which entails a considerable amount of internal assessment. A good place to start is with the practice's payer mix, the forms of payment, and the associated payment strategies. Next, conduct a review of the practice's fee schedules—an exercise that should be conducted at least annually.

Having specific knowledge of the true costs of performing various procedures and services is necessary to accomplish a comparison of acceptable fee payment associated with assigned costs. The fee (or charge master) review is followed by an assessment of the internal productivity standards, referral patterns, and compensation incentives.

Last to consider is the stability of the practice in terms of transfer of ownership, staffing, and other factors of strength.

Evaluating the Payer Mix

Preparing the practice for maximization of value involves the consideration of the *payer mix*, a frequently used term for the makeup of categories of payers. Payer mix can include self-pay, traditional or indemnity insurance, managed care organizations (MCO), and federal- and state-funded programs, such as Medicare and Medicaid. The mix of payers is immensely important to the practice; and depending on the type of practice, the payer mix can cause great variances in operating results. For example, a practice weighted heavily with Medicare patients (in which professional fees are significantly discounted) will not compare favorably in profit margins and ensuing *value* with a practice bound by fewer contractual discounts. An internal medicine practice with a payer mix that includes 50% or more Medicare and Medicaid patients, as compared with one with 35% or less, presumably will operate at lower margins, better cash flows, and lower valuation totals.

In contrast, a practice that performs a large number of elective procedures and services may not depend so heavily on third-party payments, with the presumption that these patients will be expected to pay according to the physician's fee schedule (possibly even paid as a percentage of charges). Margins, therefore, are much greater. This concept can be applied to any of the valuation methodologies to enhance practice value.

Enhancing the Payer Mix

Obtaining maximum payment relies largely on developing a strategy to enhance the payer mix. A profitable practice must maintain a desirable payer mix that includes non-discounted fees. In general, the greater the number of discounted fees, the lower the resulting valuation of the practice is. A significant strategy, as an example, would be for the practice leaders (including physicians) to visit area employers that carry certain MCO coverage, and thus market the practice's service offering to targeted employers.

The question becomes, "How will the practice moderate levels of payer mix?" Many variables influence the answer, including the following:

- The age of the physicians and their practice
- The age of physicians' patients
- Strategic alliances (as a source for patient referrals)
- The marketing strategies for the practice
- Managed care involvement
- The geographic setting (eg, urban vs rural)

The following example highlights a case in which the physician's practice profile has a significant relationship with the payer mix:

> A physician in his early 60s has practiced at the same location for more than 25 years. His patient base has not changed over time (ie, he now has minimal managed care involvement as compared to his patients' Medicare eligibility). This is typical of an internal medicine practice in which the majority of patients were pre-Medicare age at the outset. More than likely, the physician's patient base has aged with him, and now most of the patients are receiving Medicare. Their ability to pay the out-of-pocket portion may also be sensitive due to the age and work situation for the patient and family.

The ratio of Medicare patients must be considered in the valuation process as a significant factor in its operating results. To maximize practice value, the physician can pursue several options. In this example, the physician can do very little at this stage to alter the payer mix (ie, he will want to maintain the current patient population). However, even in this phase, he can improve the payer ratio by aggressively marketing to patients that make up a more favorable MCO/employer payer mix. He may achieve this through direct involvement and a concerted effort toward certain local employers whereby win-win scenarios of increased volumes at competitive prices may be accomplished. Assistance is available also for patient referrals from the hospitals where he serves as an active member of the medical staff.

As physicians see these trends developing, they can modify their payer mix. Changes are not effortless, however, and can be difficult depending on the specialty. By the nature of their specialty, internists are apt to see a high percentage of Medicare patients, and thus may not alter such payer mix significantly simply due to a practice type chosen.

Developing a Balanced Payer Mix

Developing a balanced payer mix enhances practice value for the future. Not only does this augment the value for a prospective purchaser, it also positively reflects to a managed care company reviewing and credentialing physicians for its panels. Conversely, physicians can work hard to achieve a more favorable payer mix with uncertain results, or they can do nothing and be sure of the outcome, which may not necessarily be unfavorable.

Knowledge and appreciation for the payer mix gives the owner a realistic view for the potential attraction and value of the practice and the time needed to prepare for the sale. It takes time to make changes, and typically they occur through a long-term process. Realistically, changes in payer mix cannot start in the same year that the physician prepares the practice for valuation and subsequent sale. The cycle takes three to five years prior to the sale, and even at that, a lot will depend on the practice's competitive position in the community, number and reputation of the providers, facilities, and location, and many other considerations. This concept and advice thus helps illustrate the necessity for planning constantly in a practice's lifespan in that one can never really know when the timing might be right or when a transaction decision may need to be made.

The practice owner who needs to sell within the next several years will have an opportunity to enhance value through a concerted marketing strategy and managed care campaign. The physician who needs to sell immediately, however, will have less time to achieve shifts in the payer mix, and if the valuation must be done soon, the practice's value must be considered essentially at its current level. The independent appraiser, who must be fair and objective, will be reluctant to assume significant changes in payer mix or margins in payment after the sale. Payer mix trends are a major consideration; if the trends indicate little, if any, improvements in payment in the future, the appraiser must draw conclusions accordingly.

Fee Schedule Analysis

As delineated within Chapter 1, the setting of the physician's fees and the subsequent collections influence the definitive value of the practice. Thus, it is essential to have a balance of payers to benefit the practice. Not only does this ensure that fees have been set high enough to capture the existing indemnity insurance coverage, but also it identifies the costs of providing services, while the practice ensures the coverage of costs and strives to make a profit.

Medicare

Medicare's physician fee schedule uses a relative value system known as the resource-based relative value system (RBRVS). The RBRVS is a system for measuring physician input to medical services for the purpose of calculating a physician fee schedule. The relative value of each service is the sum of relative value units (RVU) presenting physician work, practice expenses, and the cost of malpractice insurance.

The Medicare physician fee schedule amounts are adjusted to reflect the variation in practice costs from area to area. A geographic practice cost index (GPCI) has been established for every Medicare payment locality for each of the three components of a procedure's RVU (ie, the RVUs for work, practice expense, and malpractice). The GPCIs are applied in the calculation of a fee schedule payment amount by multiplying the RVU for each component times the GPCI for that component.

To understand how the Centers for Medicare and Medicaid Services (CMS) determine Medicare physician fee payments, look at the following payment formula for 2010:

$$\text{2010 pricing amount} = \left[\left(\text{Work RVU} \times \text{Work GPCI}\right) + \left(\text{Practice Expense GPCI} \times \text{Practice Expense GPCI}\right) + \left(\text{Malpractice RVU} \times \text{Malpractice GPCI}\right)\right] \times \text{Conversion Factor}$$

For example: 99213 = [(0.73 × 1.004) + (0.68 × 1.053) + (0.03 × 0.942)] × 38.215 = $56.45

The conversion factor is the multiplier that transforms relative values into payment amounts.

Managed Care Implications

An upheaval in the industry has resulted from these influences. Groups formed and hospitals bought up practices in an attempt to stay afloat in their marketplaces. The trending over the years has been cyclical. The early 1990s saw hospitals aggressively buying practices or forming physician-hospital alliances of many forms. The late 1990s and early 2000s showed a slowdown in such activity to the point of hospitals *disengaging* the purchased (employed) practices. In many cases, this meant encouraging or outright forcing the employed physician back into the community, often with hospital financial and operational support.

The current trend since around 2006 has been once again for hospitals to steer toward favorable alliances that effectively align a physician entity with its hospital system. Although many hospital practices have thrived and served their purpose well, others have been disengaged from hospitals or other integrated models due to mismanagement of competition that never materialized as originally anticipated. At any rate, the industry is still in a state of flux; physicians still want to sell their practices, either for retirement or for perhaps other financial or personal issues, including life-work balance opportunities.

A practice's ability to engage in favorable managed care arrangements has a huge effect on the value of the practice. To take advantage of favorable managed care initiatives would be another significant reason behind a decision to affiliate closely with the local health care system. Patients are often represented by large employers, insurance organizations, and MCOs seeking to contract with providers who can offer seamless health care services. These services are designed to meet most medical needs within a single integrated delivery system (IDS). Providers with more integrated medical organizations are positioning themselves now and in the future by increasing their economic viability.

Whatever the motivation for optimizing the value, physicians respond to the pressures of managed care as they relate to the sale of the practice. The current movement toward increased managed care means different things to different providers (ie, primary care vs specialty care). An understanding of the implications of managed care to each of the provider groups is required to address sufficiently the question of valuation.

Primary Care Practices

Occasionally, in working with MCOs, primary care physicians (eg, family practice, internal medicine, pediatrics, often obstetrics and gynecology) are still viewed as case managers and, therefore, the patient's first point of access to health care services. Serving in the role of coordinators of care (or gatekeepers), primary care physicians have long experienced increased responsibility and significance in the industry. However, the trend has substantially changed to the offering of high-deductible plans and the use of Health Savings Accounts (HSA), which tend to be monitored more by the employee or patient.

Plans that only offer one payment resource for a given episode of care among all providers (capitated plans as in the original example) place physicians at greater risk than traditional fee-for-service structures. The current consideration of Accountable Care Organizations (ACO) will clearly be another example of such industry evolvement. Success or failure depends on the flow of patients through the system and referral-decision process. Practice losses could result from overutilization of provider services because established fees are not increased to cover additional services under the expanded episode of care being administered. Multispecialty groups and IDS are increasingly dependent on primary care practitioners to efficiently direct patient flow through the system.

These factors contribute to why primary care physicians' practices are those most often acquired. Intangible assets of physicians play a pivotal role in the purchase price (if not the sole component), particularly when considering the managed care gatekeeper function.

The influence of managed care must be considered when the independent appraiser values the primary care practice. When calculating the value of the intangible assets, particularly post-acquisition and what contribution this practice will make to the IDS and managed care environment in the area, the appraiser must weigh the following characteristics and issues:

- Operating reputations of the practice and number of years in practice in the service area
- Local health care scenarios of managed care trends (ie, shifts from traditional payers to MCOs and health maintenance organization/preferred provider organization [HMO/PPO] penetration)
- Overall economic condition of the primary service area
- Practice's historical experience of providing service in a managed care environment

- Presence of several significant health care providers and/or payers (eg, competing hospitals, insurance companies, MCOs)
- General demographics of the practice (ie, heavily populated urban and suburban vs rural areas)

Primary care physicians are often recruited to serve on managed care panels and as sources of referrals for local hospitals. Perceived as lower cost alternatives to specialists, they typically administer a larger portion of total health care service to defined patient populations. This advances the objectives of managed care, which is to provide medical services of quality at the lowest possible cost.

Specialty Care Practices

Primary care and the role of the primary care physician as a case manager pose specific issues for specialists. Most internists serve in multiple roles: personal physicians to local patients, consultants to other physicians, and co-managing patient care with colleagues from other specialties or subspecialties.

Specialists in internal medicine often function as part of the primary care network and subsequently as coordinators of care; internists who have subspecialized can be limited to the role of a consultant. This role is communicated or presented by the way internists are listed in provider directories and in the referral mechanisms that occasionally are used to limit and control referrals from primary care physicians to consulting specialists.

Historically, specialists have been less pressured to control costs, even though they may be constrained by benefit design and utilization review criteria. Higher fees have been tolerated due to medical need and expected as compensation for extended training. Compared with other providers, specialists have commanded a disproportionately higher portion of total health care spending. As cost-containment pressures have mounted, managed care has placed emphasis on the primary care physician to regulate the use of specialists.

Due to the present environment surrounding managed care, specialists face the continued scrutiny of reduced fee-for-service arrangements, discounted pricing, and dependence on primary care practitioners for referred revenues. Specialists are concerned, and understandably so, when one considers that such a significant portion of their economic livelihood is beyond their control.

Certain considerations for intangible assets must be made for valuation of both primary care and specialty practices. In addition, the following contribute significant value to the intangible assets of specialty practices:

- The reputation and prominence of the medical specialist
- The size of the medical specialty and its correlated market share within the service area

- The supply of medical providers in that specialty in the area vs the demands for services
- The ultimate age of assets to be independently valued (fully depreciated assets can reduce overall enterprise value if replacement cost is not properly considered).

This consideration of intangible value shows the effect of managed care on both primary care and specialty practices and the value of practices. The increased emphasis on primary care physicians justifies a rise in the values of these practices (under certain market conditions). (See Chapter 9 for a review of methodologies of practice valuation, most of which depend on expectations of increased earnings and cash flows to enhance value.)

Specialty practices are generally expected to experience a decline in value as managed care continues to gain market share. The ensuing fees and limited access to patients will drive down their margins, reducing their valuation amount.

Market dynamics in the geographical service area could justify a higher valuation amount pertaining to a significant intangible asset value. The relevance and appropriateness of any level of intangible asset value of a practice transfer may only be proven through extensive analysis and understanding of the operations of the practice, area market conditions, and competition.

The knowledge and experience of qualified and independent professional appraisers are essential to ensure accuracy in the valuation, particularly relating to managed care and when valued as part of an affiliation beyond just the physician practice. Such examples of typical affiliations would include ACOs, physician hospital organizations, IDS, and joint ventures. In other words, specific valuation of the entity receiving a value calculation must be separated from the larger organization (if one indeed exists).

Productivity Standards

After assessing the external issues, such as payment through managed care and other third-party payers, the practice owner should also consider internal productivity standards. These standards relate essentially to the amount of work and volume of services rendered by the individual providers. The question of how many patient encounters and procedures can or should be performed per individual provider is significant. A popular and increasingly accepted methodology is the use of work relative value units (wRVU). This methodology often is viewed as most objective and fair to both the practice and an acquiring entity. Preparing for maximizing value would mean that the greater the individual productivity, the more likely the practice will carry a higher value. This is consistent with the methodologies that are applied to derive conclusions of fair market value.

A practice with providers who average only 5 to 10 encounters or procedures per day versus those who average 15 to 25 encounters (both statistics include surgical procedures) is more likely of lesser value. Similarly, using the example of wRVUs, if an objective source such as the Medical Group Management Association indicates a certain specialty resulted in a median position of 4,000 wRVUs and the practice under consideration for acquisition generated 3,000 wRVUs, it simply does not carry the value of a like practice with a greater amount of production.

The question the owner should ask in preparation for the sale of the practice is whether or not individual productivity can be increased. If so, then this should be used as a catalyst for improving productivity. In many instances, it may be a good idea to suspend the valuation and sale of the practice for a considerable period (eg, perhaps a year or more) to reach a level of consistent increased productivity.

The independent appraiser must also assess the productivity levels. If the appraiser cannot justifiably assume that individual productivity will improve, then it must be assumed that productivity will either stay constant or perhaps decline, especially if there are indications of such. This level of productivity will significantly affect the conclusions of value.

Whether productivity can be increased to enhance the value of the practice will depend on the unique circumstances of each practice. Some physicians will say that they simply cannot work harder or faster without compromising quality, which indeed may be the case.

Similarly, the appraiser will have to assess the realities of future productivity, although it may be difficult to consider what a new owner will produce. The appraiser's only option, therefore, is to base productivity assumptions on the current provider's performance, both historically and prospectively.

Referral Patterns

Referral patterns also serve as a significant factor in levels of individual physician productivity. Primary care physicians must work with the marketplace directly, either through managed care arrangements or by other marketing initiatives to gain access to patients. Depending on the managed care environment, specialists must depend heavily on referrals. On the other hand, the practice specialty will determine whether physicians will be able to procure patients directly without referrals. Even without the managed care factor, many patient referrals are from other physicians.

Strengthening the referral base is essential in maximizing the practice's value. For example, the appraiser must be convinced when valuing the practice that the historical referral base will be maintained, if not exceeded, under the new owner's direction. In this example, as with all cases, the first step is to make sure that the new owner will continue to garner the historical referrals, and that the referral stream will remain constant, particularly in a practice specialty that depends heavily on referrals. The seller of the practice can be very effective in keeping referral patterns strong through good service, continual feedback, and responsiveness to other professionals. It is important to keep in mind, however, that financial incentives are prohibited and are not relevant in terms of maximizing practice value.

Compensation Incentives

Another way to maintain productivity levels of the existing provider base in preparation for sale of the practice is through a well-planned and productivity-based compensation incentive model. An incentive plan model that is based on productivity is usually responsive and used quite commonly among practices to improve their overall operating margins. It is also a strategy that can be used to improve productivity in preparation for maximizing value prior to a sale. Although not part of this chapter, which specifically addresses value, it is noted that the more successful incentive compensation models include an element for a non-productivity factor. This factor would typically include a value consideration for administrative matters, required meetings and professional sessions, and initiatives of quality measurement that do not necessarily easily equate to specific productivity.

Compensation plans can be based on various measurements of productivity, including gross charges or full-fee schedule charges, net charges, net collections, number of encounters, number of surgical procedures, number of new patients, and wRVUs and total RVUs. Incentive programs used to motivate non-owner physicians to maximize productivity should always be equitable and lawful.

Provider Stability

Ensuring that revenue is maintained throughout the long term will largely depend on the stability of the providers; however, it will also depend on the strength of the support staff. Stability is the result of a good working environment; adequate support staff in terms of credentials and longevity; training and education of providers and others staff members, as appropriate; a highly rewarded, productivity-based compensation plan; a reasonable payment structure to ensure adequate funds to distribute among the providers; and sound operational management, including the essential element of a strong and creditable leader as the administrator/executive director. Practice stability is a key factor in maintaining the base of revenue, which is an outcome of having a successful referral base, along with a high level of patients, as well as referral satisfaction.

Enhancing Value through Expense Controls

As briefly addressed in Chapter 5 in preparation for selling a practice, controlling expenses is a vital topic for preparing for attaining maximum value.

Controls have two connotations in a medical practice. The first is controlling cost through careful management oversight. The second is more subtle and involves efficient operations, which inherently control expenses by supporting higher levels of productivity. An overall reason to initiate strong internal controls is to safeguard the practice's assets.

Controlling Operating Expenses

One way to increase value in the appraiser's eyes is to control operating expenses. Operating expenses can be divided into two major components: general operating and administrative overhead and cost associated specifically with all providers. General overhead includes everyday clinical and nonclinical expenses of the operation. Provider cost includes salaries, benefits, and expenses directly attributable to the physician and nonphysician providers.

In anticipation of bringing the medical practice to market and enhancing its value beforehand, the owner should review all major expense classifications, which generally consist of the following four major categories:

- Salaries and benefits
- Rent, occupancy, and other facility-related expenses
- Office and medical supply costs
- General and administrative expenses

Salaries and Benefits

The greatest single expense in the medical practice is salaries and benefits. To assess salary costs, the practice owner will need to review a list of all employees, their job descriptions, salaries, and associated benefits in the same way that the appraiser will examine them. Is the number of staff adequate? Will they fulfill their responsibilities in the best possible manner according to their job description?

Another consideration that is parallel to preparing the valuation is the employment of family members and their relative contribution. For example, some practices may employ family members who either draw a salary higher than market compensation or do not function as an employee. The owner of the practice should review this situation from an appraiser's standpoint and make the appropriate payroll adjustments in preparation for the sale of the practice. Although all changes may not need to occur immediately, identifying these situations will enable the adjustments to be made prior to the transfer of ownership.

Job descriptions are also important to consider individual credentials and resulting compensation. Long-term employees who have proven their value over time should be assured that every effort will be made to try to protect their position. Conversely, the practice may need to adjust for over- or under-qualified employees several years prior to the actual sale. By conducting a fair and objective analysis of the practice's staffing and job duties and notifying its employees of intentions to sell, the employer is showing consideration.

Benefits are also a major consideration. While some benefit expenses may be adjusted under the new ownership (which the appraiser must denote), for the most part, the benefits that are established are those that would be expected by the employees under the new ownership. An exception might be retirement plans that are replaced with a different plan, at least at the commencement of the new ownership. Most other benefits could be expected to continue.

The objective in reviewing expenses prior to the valuation is to analyze every expense for its legitimacy and necessity, particularly salaries and benefits, which generally make up approximately half of the general overhead of most practices. Adjustments should be appropriately made not just to make the bottom line look good but also as a measure of proper planning. In the end, the new owner's perspective will be different, which should be imparted at the appropriate time to the staff. (This should not initiate an overreaction nor should the staff be alarmed as a result of preparation to sell the practice).

Administrative Overhead

Evaluation of all other sources of administrative overhead should follow the consideration of personnel expense. Industry statistics and benchmarks should be used as a comparison as these are evaluated, preparing the practice for valuation and, ultimately, its sale. Adjustments should occur where warranted, taking care not to cut out necessary operational expenses, just the individual line items that could be viewed as exorbitant or unnecessary.

This logic follows with each of the other major areas of general overhead, including rent and facility expenses, general administrative expenses, and supply commitments.

Rental rate and space may be difficult to adjust in the case of a long-term lease. The practice owner who is also the owner of the facility must decide whether to sell the real estate or lease it to the new owner. (The real estate is rarely part of the practice review and valuation. It is and should be a separate legal entity subject to its own independent valuation.)

Thus, the rent should be considered in the context of who the owner or lessor shall be after the sale. For example, if the dermatologist owner of the practice is also the owner of the real estate, including the building, then a new lease can easily be consummated with the new owner of the practice. If there are other owners of the building, it is possible that a new lease may be negotiated or, at the very least, the existing lease assigned or sublet under the same terms and conditions of the existing lease. From a preplanning aspect, it depends on what the terms of the lease will be and who the lessor will be after the sale.

In ownership, there could be some flexibility in rental rate. Conversely, for the most part, everyone (no matter whom the lessor is) will want to obtain a fair and equitable market rate for the property. The current rent at market rates should be determined as an aspect of planning. For various internal reasons, the rent may be on the higher side of fair market value on some occasions (eg, when the dermatologist owner of the practice also owns the real estate). This may need to be adjusted to appeal to a new owner of the practice to lease the facilities, which is a matter to be considered by both the physician and the appraiser when preparing for the valuation. Rent believed to be significantly under or over market value will be adjusted in the valuation calculations, particularly under an income approach.

In general, cost containment should be an overriding principle, whether the practice is ongoing or being prepared for valuation and subsequent sale. Figure 13-1 illustrates general overhead categories that should be considered and controlled prior to completion of the valuation.

Salaries and Benefits—Staff

Insurance—Business and Professional

Supplies—Medical

Supplies—Office

Travel and Entertainment

Repairs and Maintenance

Occupancy Costs

Depreciation Expense

Interest Expense

FIGURE 13-1 General Overhead Categories

Physician Compensation and Benefits

Perhaps the greatest expense is provider compensation and benefits. Compensation is simply a result of the monies left over after all other expenses are paid in practices in which ownership is shared by the physicians and no providers are employees. Employed providers are usually paid using a combination of salary and incentive bonus. Planning for valuation and sale or merger calls for consideration of these historical compensation figures, as it is a major factor within the valuation process. The independent appraiser must consider and render an opinion about the stability and viability of the provider base, which may include the current owners' knowledge of likely change in ownership, or their potential for exiting the practice, subject to the sale. An additional factor that an independent appraiser must exhibit is the age of each provider. If a prospective buyer sees the opportunity for market (or above-market) compensation after the acquisition, and this is substantiated in the valuation analysis, the prospects of a sale increase immensely.

Enhancing Value through Strategic Planning

Strategic planning—a commonly overused term—should be of significance to the practice. A successful plan for the future, considering organizing principles in key areas, is crucial both for the practice that is contemplating sale or merger and for continued operations under the same ownership. A beneficial strategic plan considers organizing principles in the following six key areas:

1. Patients
2. Technical skills
3. Administrative skills
4. Support skills
5. Alliances
6. Divestures (areas of business that will not be sought out or accepted, or after analysis are indicated to be of lesser value to the new entity)

All businesses need a blueprint for action, or a strategic plan. Each plan will vary with the present issues of the organization. A medical practice being contemplated for a sale or merger will differ significantly from one that is being planned to continue under current ownership for the foreseeable future. The important point is to have a plan for the future. First, a plan is necessary to achieve and maintain stability. Second, a strategic plan offers a significant advantage in the search for a partner or purchaser if the practice is to be sold or merged with another practice.

The busier the practice (more services and locations, number of providers), the more useful the strategic plan. Long-term planning in key areas is important regardless of whether the practice is up for sale or in the process of transition.

Several strategic questions and issues should be asked and considered when preparing the practice for sale or merger. They include the following:

- What is the nature of the practice and the services that are performed?
- How do regulatory forces influence its operations both now and in the future?
- Are there any significant services that will be changed due to the economy, regulatory matters, or other external issues?
- What effect does the future of electronic communications and data gathering have on the practice (including electronic health record initiatives)?
- What are some of the education standards and their effect on staffing (both clinical and nonclinical, provider and nonprovider)?
- What is the geographic range of the practice and where are the future opportunities or challenges relative to this? The practice owners should ensure their knowledge of both their respective primary service area and the properly defined secondary service area. This must be performed by an independent and creditable source.
- What emerging practices are in this area that would provide specific competition (eg, the presence of another similar practice or other specialty that does some similar procedures)?
- What capabilities does the practice have for meeting the demands of competition?
- Who are the key sources of patients (primary providers and third-party payers)?
- How dependent is the practice on keeping these patients (likely represented by certain large payers)?
- Who are the key third-party payers in the practice's service area that are not served by the practice?
- What is the scope of clinical resources and challenges of the practice?
- Does the practice use information technology and specialized staff to leverage professional expertise?
- How are the practice's services marketed and to what extent should they be communicated to the community?
- Who has responsibility for future development of the products and services within the practice?

Identification of strategic issues is a critical part of planning and is important, even if the practice is contemplating new ownership. To the potential new owner, a strategic plan ensures that the practice is an ongoing, viable, sustaining entity and helps the independent appraiser assess the practice's growth potential. It could even increase the value of the practice under the income approach through more aggressive, yet justified, growth projections.

Thus, setting a strategic plan for the practice in preparation for sale or merger is important. Strategic planning sets out the following major areas:

- Identifying the practice's capabilities
- Determining future opportunities
- Establishing goals
- Establishing priorities
- Developing a clear plan to realize the results desired for the future

Part of the strategic plan may be the sale or merger of the practice, which is not necessarily a negative in the context of the overall process under consideration. In fact, most prospective buyers should be impressed by the fact that the existing owners have thought through their situation enough to conclude a possible sale or merger as a part of their ongoing strategic initiatives. Other basic considerations and questions in strategic planning include:

- Who are we? How does the community perceive us? How does the provider (especially primary care) community perceive us?
- Where are we today? At what stage in our practice maturity cycle do we view ourselves?
- How do we want to conduct ourselves? How should we appear to the community?
- Where are we going? How best to illustrate and communicate that?
- How are we going to get to where we want to go? Do we publish a plan?
- What is the best way to measure our progress?
- Do we need a major change in ownership to accomplish our goals and objectives? (This component requires honest and thorough self-evaluation to implement needed changes).

In addition, it is also good for the practice to define its mission and values, typically through periodically updated statements that clarify the practice's vision for the future.

An environmental assessment that reviews the widest range of factors that influence the practice's operations and breaks them down into various concerns for the future should follow. This assessment could include economic, social, technological, regulatory, and political forces that affect the profession.

Usually, the environmental assessment calls for a strengths, weaknesses, opportunities, and threats (SWOT) analysis as an important part of the inward review of the practice and consideration of its strategic issues. The SWOT analysis should include a frank look at the providers and the services that those individuals deliver and be objective and practical in nature, realizing that there are limitations to the practice's performance results.

Thus, the practice should be thoroughly prepared for a dramatic change in the future (eg, any change in ownership) through effective strategic planning and direction. Otherwise, it is less likely to sell, and the independent appraiser's understanding of the practice's plans for the future is compromised. This concept is particularly essential as this practice is compared for valuation and subsequent acquisition with other like practices or opportunities.

Personnel Policies and Procedures Manual

Value is maximized by having sound personnel policies in place. Every practice should have a personnel policy and procedure manual. This is a simple booklet stating policies, benefits, and other protocols. The book should answer what are the guidelines and rules by which the services of a practice are administered. Such resources, although subjective, say a lot about the management of the practice. While an appraiser will not place great emphasis in this area when deriving value, having access to the policy and procedure manual that establishes the operations of the practice may positively affect the valuation to some degree. It is a great indication that this practice has been well managed.

Conclusion

The focus of this chapter has been on the components that must be considered when selling a practice. These considerations show how value can be enhanced through a number of operational initiatives. The valuation process must review each of these facets within the operations of the practice and relate them to the calculations. It must also conduct a subjective overview of the work being completed to derive, in the opinion of the appraiser, the fair market value of the medical practice. If the practice is strong and institutes sound operational systems, the practice will have greater value in the eyes of a potential purchaser.

CHAPTER 14

Fair Market Value Opinions in Physician-Hospital Compensation Relationships

OUTLINE

As the health care industry continues to evolve, so do the relationships between hospitals and physicians. Not only are increasing numbers of physician-hospital relationships emerging, but also different structures and forms of relationships are developing. Regardless of the scope or structure of the physician-hospital relationship, it is imperative that any compensation shared between the parties remain within fair market value (FMV) limitations. This chapter examines the different compensatory arrangements that currently exist between physicians and hospitals, and the regulations that govern these relationships.

Overview of Physician-Hospital Compensation Situations

During the early 1990s, there was tremendous growth in physician employment by hospitals. A significant number of physicians elected to sell their practice to a hospital and to become employed. Many of these relationships were incredibly lucrative for the physicians, and included a large amount of up-front cash for their practice (including payment for goodwill and other intangibles) coupled with high guaranteed salaries, the potential for incentive compensation based on relatively limited quality or outcome considerations, little to no risk sharing, and limited productivity expectations. Due to the financial pressures that were placed on hospitals because of these types of transactions, many of these relationships were relatively short-lived and were dissolved by the end of the decade.

Both physicians and hospitals learned a number of key lessons from this foray into alignment, and one principal lesson was that any relationship between hospitals and physicians needed to be economically viable, not only in the short term, but also over the long term. This meant that an appropriate compensation model was needed, one that accounted for the structure of the relationship, as well as the actual services being performed. A second key learning point that resulted from the 1990s boom in employment (and the subsequent dissolution of many of these agreements) was that employment was not the only structure that physicians and hospitals could use to create an ongoing relationship between them.

Today, numerous other relationships are considered viable, even though they stop short of full employment. At present, a spectrum of alignment options exists, ranging from limited to moderate to full forms of integration (see Figure 14-1 for further information regarding potential forms of alignment). Employment and some forms of professional services agreements are categorized as full alignment, while other structures, such as compensation for unassigned emergency department call coverage and joint venturing, are considered limited to moderate forms of integration, respectively.

Limited Integration	Moderate Integration	Full Integration
■ *Managed Care Networks:* Loose alliances for contracting purposes ■ *Call Coverage Stipends:* Pay for unassigned Emergency Department call ■ *Medical Directorships:* Specific clinical oversight duties ■ *Gain Sharing:* Economic benefits for hospitals and physicians; isolated and targeted initiatives	■ *Service Line Management:* Management of all specialty services within the hospital ■ *MSO/ISO:* Ties hospitals to physician's business ■ *Equity Group Assimilation:* Ties entities via legal agreement; joint practice ownership ■ *Joint Ventures:* Unites parties under common enterprise; difficult to structure; legal hurdles ■ *Co-management:* Strong economic and strategic alignment; relatively minor return	■ *Employment:* Strongest alignment; minimizes economic risk for physicians ■ *Employment "Lite":* Professional services agreements (PSA) and other similar models (such as the practice management arrangement)—self-employed independent contractor

MSO: management services organizations ; ISO: information services organization

FIGURE 14-1 Types of Alignment Relationships

As opposed to the 1990s, when the physician-hospital relationship involved very little true *partnering*, the new wave of alignment options includes a singular emphasis on partnership, including a unified focus on quality of patient care, delivery of services, and cost-effective management. In addition, there is a greater emphasis on establishing reasonable economic terms for each alignment situation. Now, when physicians are employed, little, if any, intangible value is paid to the physicians. Tangible assets are paid at FMV, and a focus is on productivity-based compensation. Even under the limited to moderate forms of alignment, the compensation provided to physicians is based on the actual services performed, often as documented in timesheets that record the number of hours worked and the duties completed during this time. Compensation then is based on the actual hours worked, rather than a fixed amount, regardless of the services completed.

Overall, the current physician-hospital compensation relationships have a different look and feel than those that came into effect in the 1990s. There is a significantly greater focus on appropriate levels of compensation and additional emphasis on creating a correlation between compensation and production.

Concepts of Fair Market Value Remuneration

The FMV is an important standard of value considered when valuing a business entity (ie, a private practice). However, the concept of FMV also applies to compensation in a physician-hospital relationship.

Some of the most prevalent definitions of FMV within health care are found in the regulations for the Stark law (discussed further in Chapter 12), as well as the Internal Revenue Service (IRS) definition of FMV (discussed further in Chapter 8). When considering these definitions, one of the most significant aspects in determining FMV, in terms of compensation, is taken from the Stark law, which infers that any compensation provided to a physician should be equivalent to the compensation paid to other physicians for similar services. This is the very basis for FMV: ensuring that compensation to a physician(s) within a specific market mirrors other compensation within that same market for the same type of services, including the amount of time spent and the deliverables (or outcomes) of these services.

Another significant component relative to FMV is the disregard for the volume or value of the physician's referrals. Thus, it is important that the compensation provided to any physician is for actual work performed; otherwise, it could be considered an inducement for referrals. While this is important regardless of the alignment structure, it is particularly important in compensatory relationships with private practice physicians (as opposed to employed physicians), who have seemingly more options relative to the direction of their referrals.

Recently, several medical directorship arrangements were brought into question by the federal government, largely because limited services were provided by a physician, but a significant level of compensation was paid. Because there did not appear to be a correlation between services rendered and compensation, the relationship was further analyzed to determine whether it was actually a payment for physician referrals. Thus, to avoid even the appearance of impropriety, it is important that any compensation be based on actual work performed.

Factors Determining FMV

In determining FMV, a number of factors must be considered. The first is the scope of services to be provided. Does the physician-hospital relationship require 4 hours of work per week or 20 hours per week? The time spent delivering services will have an impact on the FMV of the transaction. A second consideration concerns the duties and responsibilities of the services provided. For example, provision of administrative services can have a different FMV than clinical, patient-care services.

Next, the specialty of the physician performing the services will affect FMV. Because of the complexity of care provided and the differing levels of compensation historically earned, a cardiologist may be compensated at a higher rate than a family practitioner for a similar breadth of services. In addition, the geographic market where the services are provided may influence the FMV. For example, FMV may vary in urban versus rural settings, in the Southeast compared to the Northeast, and in Wisconsin as compared to California.

Finally, when establishing FMV, both the amount of compensation and the manner in which it is paid should be considered. Most physician-hospital compensatory relationships that include a limited number of hours base payment on an annual, per diem, or hourly basis. While incentive compensation (ie, bonuses) may also be used, this form of compensation is typically in addition to (rather than a replacement for) a more structured form of compensation (such as an hourly payment). For compensatory relationships involving a significant number of hours (such as employment or a professional services agreement [PSA] model), remuneration may be variable, and based on production metrics such as a payment per patient encounter or per work relative value unit (wRVU) produced, rather than a fixed amount.

It is critical that any compensation within a physician-hospital relationship remains within FMV limitations. Otherwise, financial and other consequences may be levied against all involved parties under the anti-kickback statute, Stark law, IRS intermediate sanctions rules, the Federal False Claims Act, or other regulations. Therefore, it is important that physicians and hospitals recognize and abide by all applicable FMV regulations.

Commercially Reasonable Considerations

Commercial reasonableness is another factor that must be considered as part of a compensatory relationship between hospitals and physicians. Just because a transaction is considered FMV, it does not mean that it is commercially reasonable.

In assessing physician compensation, both FMV and commercial reasonableness must be considered. As it is important that both qualifications are met, many consider the terms interchangeable. However, the two concepts are distinct. The following example may better illustrate the difference between the two concepts:

An orthopedic surgeon decides to leave a solo practice to become employed by a hospital. Prior to employment, the physician's historical compensation averaged $350,000 per year. The physician's historical compensation is relatively low in comparison to industry benchmarks, even though his production was relatively high. On employment by the hospital, the physician's go-forward compensation was estimated at $700,000 per year. While the proposed compensation is more in line with a highly productive orthopedic surgeon (such as this physician), a two-fold increase in compensation may not be commercially reasonable in the physician's market, particularly if it is significantly greater than what any other employed physician (including other orthopedic surgeons) are being compensated. Thus, while this relationship may pass the test of FMV, it would not be viewed as commercially reasonable.

Use of Industry Standards and Benchmarks

A number of physician compensation surveys exist within the health care industry and serve as valuable tools for benchmarking compensation. As such, these surveys are also often a point of reference in determining FMV and commercially reasonable limitations. For academic settings, the most prevalent survey for physician compensation is that published by the American Association of Medical Colleges (AAMC).[1] To benchmark compensation for physicians in clinical practice, the Medical Group Management Association (MGMA),[2] the American Medical Group Association (AMGA),[3] and Sullivan, Cotter and Associates, Inc (SCA)[4] surveys are often considered. The MGMA, SCA, and AMGA surveys are widely recognized industry surveys, and both the MGMA and SCA surveys are approved for use by the Office of Inspector General (OIG).

In addition to surveys that publish benchmarks relative to physicians' total annual compensation, there are surveys that specialize in benchmarking compensation specific to medical directorship agreements, compensated call arrangements, and other hospital-physician relationships. Both MGMA[5] and SCA[6] publish surveys relative to administrative and call compensation; these surveys can offer greater insight into potential compensation for these specific transactions.

The physician compensation surveys typically publish benchmarks across a range of percentiles and relative to a number of criteria. For example, the MGMA survey publishes data from the 10th to the 90th percentile, in single percentile increments. Physician compensation increases across the percentiles; thus, higher compensation is associated with a higher percentile (such as the 90th percentile), while lower compensation is associated with a lower percentile (such as the 10th percentile). Many of the surveys also publish the mean (ie, the average) compensation.

These surveys also typically classify data among several variables. For example, among other variables, the AMGA survey includes benchmarks for different geographic regions (eg, Eastern, Western, Southern, and Northern); the SCA survey publishes compensation for varying physician positions (eg, staff physician, medical director or division chief, and department chair); the MGMA survey provides separate data for hospital-owned practices and non-hospital-owned practices. The multiple variations of data that exist within each of these surveys add value to the survey, as very specific information can be retrieved across a host of metrics.

Depending on the nature of the hospital-physician relationship, these surveys can be an invaluable tool in helping to establish FMV and commercial reasonableness limitations.

Process of Evaluating Work Objectives of the Physicians and Corresponding Compensation

A hospital and physician should establish well-defined compensation objectives as they prepare to forge a relationship together. The objectives should be tailored to the individual conditions of their relationship (thus, the objectives will likely vary across different hospital-physician relationships). During negotiations, both the hospital and physician will benefit by using an objective checklist (similar to the following) to derive a fair and equitable compensation plan.

- Provide compensation that is commensurate with area norms and competitive in the marketplace
- Attract top physicians
- Retain those physicians currently employed by (or otherwise aligned with) the organization
- Offer a base salary to provide income security
- Establish financial incentives to promote physician productivity and the efficiency of practice locations
- Maintain the financial viability of the organization
- Establish an objective methodology for calculating physician compensation
- Promote the sharing of risk between the physicians and the organization
- Encourage efficient and appropriate patient care
- Establish work standards for physician productivity and efficiency
- Design a compensation plan that is easy to administer
- Recognize the different incentives in capitation and fee-for-service

- Provide a mechanism for performance measurement and response for the physicians
- Distribute bonuses to physicians quarterly
- Promote a long-term commitment between the physicians and the organization
- Promote physician involvement and contributions to the organization

In addition to establishing compensation objectives at the outset of a hospital-physician relationship, it is also important to evaluate work objectives prior to finalizing an alignment transaction. This is true because the work to be completed can affect the corresponding compensation within the transaction. When determining the appropriate level of compensation for a physician, the first consideration is typically the scope of the relationship. For example, in limited forms of integration (such as medical directorships), there are likely relatively fewer responsibilities and a narrower scope of services offered by the physicians. Thus, compensation should be commensurate with this scope.

A second consideration is the complexity of the duties associated with the relationship. For example, if the physician is engaged to provide highly specialized services (such as nephrolithotripsy for pediatric patients with kidney stones), the position may warrant higher levels of compensation.

A third consideration is the availability of physicians to perform the requested services. For example, services provided to a hospital by a physician in a high-need specialty (ie, one in which a shortage of physicians exists, such as general surgery) can warrant different compensation than services provided by a specialist in more ready supply. Due to a limited supply of physicians in the specialty, a relationship with such a physician may warrant higher levels of compensation. Therefore, the scope and complexity of the work objectives can influence compensation, as can the availability of physicians who can meet the established objectives.

Outcomes-based Compensation

Another interesting consideration relative to work objectives and corresponding compensation is the potential for compensation to be based on specific, previously established outcomes. As quality and cost-sharing programs grow in popularity, so do compensation arrangements based on these outcomes. As mentioned previously, not all compensation in hospital-physician relationships must be based on a fixed amount; some relationships can have a variable level of compensation available based on attainment of specific, measurable outcomes.

For example, a recent OIG opinion[7] validated the use of variable compensation in a compensation arrangement between a hospital and a group of physicians who were jointly participating in a pay-for-performance program. The compensation, which was determined on a per capita basis, was commensurate with the achievement of defined quality objectives. The OIG concluded that this compensation structure was appropriate because it was tied to actual services provided and documented, and the method of compensation did not reward any form of fraud or abuse. Thus, variable compensation is an appropriate structure as long as it relates to the work objectives (in this case, quality objectives) that are mutually established by the physician and hospital.

Professional Services Agreement and Employment "Lite"

While the 1990s were shaped by physician employment agreements, the current decade may come to be known as the professional services agreement (PSA) era. The PSA model is a form of full integration that has many characteristics of the employment model but stops significantly short of employment in various ways. Under the PSA structure, a hospital would engage physicians to provide services for a specific service line. This would include the provision of specialty services, clinical management and coordination, service line management, medical directorships and administrative, supervisory, teaching, and research functions. The PSA model generally requires the physicians to provide services at the hospital on a full-time basis, and usually with some level of exclusivity.

There are many variants of the PSA structure, but four of the most common are:

- Hospital contracts with a practice for global payment; practice retains all management responsibilities
- Hospital employs physicians; the practice entity is retained and contracts with the hospital for administrative management; the staff are not employed by the hospital
- Hospital contracts with physicians for professional services; hospital employs staff and "owns" the administrative structure
- Hospital employs or contracts with physicians; practice entity spun-off into a jointly-owned management services organization or information services organization

While each of these four structures are viable hospital-physician relationships, we consider herein the specifics of the first PSA model cited (the global payment model) in greater depth. (Also see Figure 14-2 for further information relative to this model.)

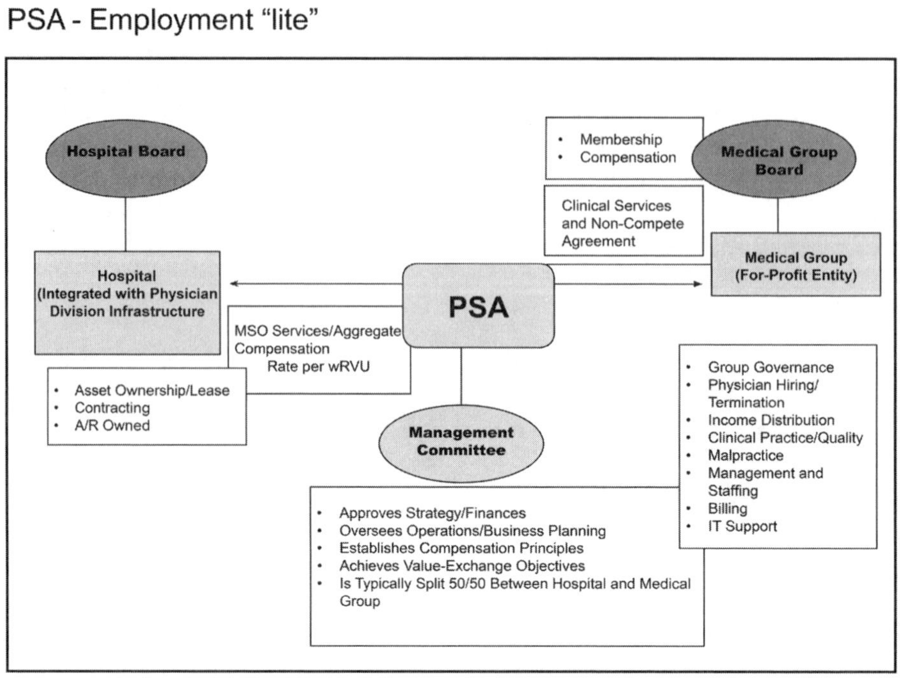

FIGURE 14-2 Diagram of Professional Services Agreement Model

Global Payment Model

Within the global payment PSA structure, the practice is an independent contractor of the hospital, and the physicians remain employees of their practice. The practice then invoices the hospital for the actual services rendered by the physicians, including clinical, diagnostic, and ancillary services. The practice remains solely responsible for all of its overhead expenses (the hospital assumes no responsibility for any operating expenses).

In exchange for services rendered, the hospital compensates the practice at FMV and commercially reasonable rates. Payment often is based on wRVU production, which quantifies the amount of services provided by the physicians in a standard, objective manner. Payment based on wRVUs is also advantageous to the physicians, as it provides payment regardless of patients' payer status. Under the global payment model, the payment per wRVU not only provides compensation to the physicians for the professional component of the clinical services rendered, it also accounts for the overhead expenses within the practice. Thus, the payment from the hospital is "global" in that it covers both operating (ie, "above the line") expenses as well as physician compensation ("below the line" expenses). (*Above the line* and *below the line* refer to the location of expenses on a practice's income statement; also often referred to as a profit and loss statement.)

Compensation and Reimbursement

On execution of the PSA, the hospital establishes the fees that the physicians are to charge for professional services. The hospital will also be responsible for negotiating the payer contracts for these services. This arrangement is typically advantageous, in that hospitals are often able to negotiate more lucrative payer contracts than individual practices. Finally, the hospital will own the accounts receivable for services rendered after the PSA model is implemented (the practice will continue to own the receivables for services rendered prior to that date).

As the practice will have retained its billing staff, the staff will typically perform the billing and collections functions related to the physicians' services in the name of the hospital, under its tax identification and billing number. As receivables are collected, they belong to the hospital. In exchange for these billing and collection services, the hospital must compensate the practice (at FMV rates); such payment generally is established as a percentage of collections.

One of the more significant aspects of the PSA model is the practice's ability to sell or lease their ancillary services to the hospital (at FMV rates). This is particularly desirable for specialties such as cardiology, for which reimbursement for ancillary services is significantly greater for the hospital than it is for a private practice as a result of recent changes in reimbursement for ancillary services such as nuclear and echocardiographic studies. The hospital bills for ancillary services under hospital outpatient department (HOPD) rates, which are greater than the rates the practice is able to receive. While the increased revenue from ancillary services cannot be paid directly to the physicians for compliance reasons, it can be used to fund the physicians' overall compensation package under this model.

The ancillaries could be left in the practice and become a part of a joint venture arrangement. But, as alluded to here, that may not provide the level of reimbursement desired. (There are very specific regulations and requirements for hospital-based ancillaries—in terms of their ownership, presentation to the public, and separation from the private practice—to be designated as "hospital-based.") Overall, an advantage of this structure (the PSA model) is for the opportunities to increase and enhance the overall bottom-line, which ultimately is the physicians' compensation.

The benefits of a PSA relationship include the following:

- Provides many of the goals of employment without such
- Physicians maintain independence from the hospital
- Practice is maintained as a single operating entity

- Management and oversight of staff remains within the practice
- Flexibility in structure
- No loss of autonomy
- Can continue all services currently provided
- Opportunities to increase and enhance bottom line for both the hospital and the practice
- Bonus opportunities for exceptional performance
- Stability in relationship with the hospital
- Opportunities to expand services together without being fully aligned (ie, employment)
- Easy segue to full employment

Historical Compensation as a Basis for Remuneration

There is an old adage that the past provides the best indicator of how the future will unfold, and this saying has some applicability to physician compensation. Specifically, historical compensation is typically one consideration in determining appropriate "go-forward" physician compensation. It is important to note, however, that historical compensation does not always reflect actual services provided. For example, in a private practice setting, a shareholder physician may experience higher compensation based on the productivity of non-shareholder physicians. Going forward, the shareholder physician's historical compensation would not serve as an appropriate representation of the work completed by that physician, and thus, should not be a driving factor for go-forward compensation.

Relative Value Units and Other Bases of Productivity

As discussed in Chapter 1, relative value units (RVUs) are used to measure productivity. The units are based on standards established by the resource-based relative value scale (RBRVS), which Medicare began using in 1992. The RVUs measure complexity or severity by taking into account the physician's effort, stress, judgment, and other qualities that are required to perform a specific procedure. They establish the value of one service relative to another. For example, a simple office visit has a lower RVU than a surgical procedure. Each procedure is considered in terms of the following three components to obtain relative value:

- Work
- Practice operations
- Malpractice expense

The RVU is "payer blind," in that the same RVU weight is assigned regardless of a patient's payer classification. Use of RVUs eliminates fee schedule variances for the same service. They also eliminate the need to differentiate between gross and net charges. RVUs are becoming the standards of productivity, more so than other, traditional measures of production such as:

- Gross charges
- Collections
- Patient visits
- Hospital encounters
- Surgery cases
- Articles published (typically only applied in an academic setting)

Given their growing acceptance within the industry as the principal measure of physician productivity, many compensation models are beginning to use RVUs. Specifically, work-only RVUs (wRVUs) have become the primary measure of production, as this component accounts for the actual work performed by the physician, without consideration of any financial aspects (such as overhead or malpractice). Within a compensation plan, wRVUs are converted to dollars through a derivative called a conversion factor. A simplified physician compensation calculation follows, along with an example of the calculation in use (see Figure 14-3):

$$\text{Total wRVUs} \times \text{Conversion Factor} = \text{Physician Compensation}$$

Total wRVUs are determined by individual productivity. The conversion factor is determined by external benchmarks or internally established budgets or benchmarks.

As noted in Figure 14-3, the accumulated wRVUs are converted based on a $24 per wRVU conversion factor. The resulting physician compensation is the conversion factor times the total number of wRVUs produced.

Several factors need to be considered when transitioning to or implementing a wRVU system for compensation. The first is the reality of transferring productivity in the form of wRVUs to actual "dollars and cents." This conversion requires a thorough analysis to ensure that neither too little nor too much compensation is being provided. When converting such monies to comparatives from one specialty to another, the legitimacy of the overall wRVU conversion factor should be thoroughly analyzed.

Second, the realization that a wRVU-based system does not reward any behaviors other than raw productivity should be understood. There are some ways to address this. For example, many compensation plans introduce a nonproductivity-based pool that assigns an additional dollar

CPT Code	CPT Description	Units of Service Provided by Physician	wRVU*	Result
99211	Established patient, office, or other outpatient	550	0.52	286.00
99212	Established patient, office, or other outpatient	415	0.94	390.10
99213	Established patient, office, or other outpatient	3,057	1.32	4,035.24
99214	Established patient, office, or other outpatient	1,045	2.06	2,152.70
99215	Established patient, office, or other outpatient	150	3.06	459.00
Total wRVUs generated by physician over last 12 months				7,323.04
Sample conversion factor†				× $24.00
Resulting Physician Compensation				$175,752.96

* This is based on work relative value units (wRVU)

† Not the Medicare conversion factor

FIGURE 14-3 Simplified Physician Compensation Calculation

amount to be distributed based on the physicians' performance relative to an overall attitude of expense control. Transitioning to a wRVU-based compensation system is a four-step process:

1. Organize a transition team.
2. Compare practice-specific current procedural terminology (CPT®) codes with the wRVU schedules.
3. Design and develop a wRVU-based report.
4. Analyze wRVU production data.

Figure 14-4 presents schedules that summarize examples of three reports and the appropriate formula that should be used. The reports include the following:

- Example Service of RVU for Office Outpatient Visit (CPT® Code 99213)
- Simplified Physician Compensation Calculation
- wRVU Report Format

Example Service of wRVU for Office Outpatient Visit (CPT Code 99213)

Component	Description	wRVU
Work	Physician resources, including time, stress, skill, physical and mental effort, and judgment	0.67
Practice	Operating costs of the medical practice	0.69
Malpractice	Professional liability expense	0.03
Total RVU		1.39

Simplified Physician Compensation Calculation

CPT Code	CPT Description	Units of Service Provided by Physician	wRVU*	Result
99211	Established patient, office, or other outpatient	550	0.17	93.50
99212	Established patient, office, or other outpatient	415	0.45	186.75
99213	Established patient, office, or other outpatient	3,057	0.67	2048.19
99214	Established patient, office, or other outpatient	1,045	1.10	1149.5
99215	Established patient, office, or other outpatient	150	1.77	265.50
	Total wRVUs generated by physician over last 12 months			3743.44
	Sample conversion factor†			× $36.1992
	Resulting Physician Compensation			$135,509.53

* This is based on work relative value units (wRVU)

† Not the Medicare conversion factor

wRVU Report Format

Service Code	Month-to-Date Units	Year-to-Date Units	wRVU	Month-to-Date wRVUs	Year-to-Date wRVUs	Conversion Factor	Month-to-Date Compensation	Year-to-Date Compensation
99211	46	550	0.17	7.82	93.5	36.1992	$283.07	$3,384.62
99212	35	415	0.45	15.72	186.75	36.1992	$569.05	$6,760.20
99213	225	3,057	0.67	150.72	2048.19	36.1992	$5,457.03	$74,142.84
99214	87	1,045	1.1	95.7	1149.5	36.1992	$3,464.26	$41,610.98
99215	13	150	1.77	23.01	265.5	36.1992	$832.94	$9,610.89
Total				**292.97**	**3,743.44**	**36.1992**	**$10,346.35**	**$135,509.53**

Formula: Total wRVUs × Conversion Factor = Physician Compensation

Note: Total wRVUs are determined by individual productivity. Conversion factor is external benchmarks or internally established budgets or benchmarks

FIGURE 14-4 Transitioning to a Work Relative Value Unit System

Expense Considerations Relative to Physician-Hospital Compensation and FMV/Commercially Reasonable Opinions

In many physician-hospital alignment strategies, the hospital's overall relationship with a physician results in a net loss to the hospital (ie, the revenue generated as a result of the relationship is less than the expenses incurred). This situation is especially true in physician employment arrangements in which the hospital must operate the practice and provide the physician with FMV compensation and benefits. For example, the loss per year can be as high as $50,000 to $125,000 per employed primary care physician.

Neither of the compensation guiding principles (ie, FMV and commercial reasonableness limitations) prohibits a hospital from realizing a net loss as a result of their physician alignment strategy, but these losses must be within acceptable limitations. For example, a hospital cannot incur a net loss of $500,000 for a pediatrician because it opted to compensate that physician $450,000 (clearly outside the boundaries of market compensation for a physician within that specialty). This said, hospitals and physicians should work together to create an understandable and fiscally sound compensation plan.

Within a compensation plan, the hospital's goal is to exercise sound business reasoning before committing to a physician compensation package that is relevant to the economic and legal constraints present. In a private practice, typically, operating expenses consume 50% or more of revenue. The remaining 50% (or a lesser amount) remains available for use as physician compensation (including benefits and incentive pay).

The physicians' goal is to attain a compensation package that is comparable to (or slightly greater than) their current total income. For example, physicians who are anticipating selling their practice and becoming employees want to maintain (or ideally increase) their income level. When physicians own and operate their own practice, they have to work and produce to manage their business. Their income is based on any excess over collections and expenses. As employees, ordinarily, they are guaranteed a base compensation by the employer that does not depend on the success or failure of the practice. Income simply depends on the physicians' adherence to the employment contract. The objective is to make up the difference or exceed current income with an incentive provision.

The goals of a physician compensation plan, which should be reviewed constantly while formulating the relationship and even after its implementation, are as follows:

- Develop a logical, economically supportable basis of measuring and compensating production

- Consider overall profitability (including cost savings) of the relationship as a criterion for determining compensation
- Consider patient satisfaction as a measurement standard of performance and, ultimately, compensation
- Encourage the physician to be a team player (part of a larger health care delivery system), not just an independent practitioner or entrepreneur
- Reward successful performance and penalize poor performance

Conclusion

As a result of recent (and anticipated) changes in the health care industry, the number of physician-hospital relationships is increasing. Physicians in particular are looking to align with hospitals, who can offer much-needed support and stability in the wake of a rapidly changing environment. Current hospital-physician relationships range from limited forms of integration (such as medical directorships or call compensation) to full forms of integration (such as employment or a PSA model), and include many different variants and hybrid models. Regardless of the relationship, however, one fact remains constant: it is imperative that any compensation between physicians and hospitals falls within FMV and commercial reasonableness limitations. While, typically, an independent valuator is needed to determine FMV and commercially reasonable limitations, physicians and hospitals can consider two practical rules as they contemplate potential compensation structures and amounts:

- If it seems too good to be true, it likely is.
- If it is more complicated than you can understand, it needs simplifying.

First, if a relationship includes a long term (ie, anything longer than eight years), a large amount of guaranteed compensation, potential for generous incentive compensation, and little risk, it is more likely that the government will consider this transaction noncompliant. Second, if the structure of the relationship and the corresponding compensation includes a great deal of complexity, it may need restructuring. While not all agreements need to follow the same structure, the more unusual a relationship is (including its formula for physician payment), the more attention it will likely raise. Generally, a simple yet effective relationship can meet the needs of all parties and avoid the pitfalls that come with transactions that are more complicated.

In summary, a number of legal and regulatory requirements govern hospital-physician relationships, and all of these must be considered when formulating an alignment structure, particularly one that involves compensation. The federal government is beginning to take closer notice of physician compensation arrangements, and is more strictly enforcing the rules and regulations relative to these arrangements. Therefore, it is important that hospitals and physicians protect themselves by engaging exclusively in compensation arrangements that are within FMV limitations.

Endnotes

1. *Report on Medical School Faculty Salaries 2009–2010.* Washington, DC: Association of American Medical Colleges; 2011.
2. *Physician Compensation and Production Survey: 2011.* Englewood, CO: Medical Group Management Association; 2010.
3. Vaudrey BSJ, Loos SJ. Compensation 2010: Emerging models, shifting priorities. Results from the AMGA 2010 Medical Group Compensation and Financial Survey. *Group Prac J* September 2010;11–18.
4. *2010 Physician Compensation and Productivity Survey.* Atlanta, GA: Sullivan, Cotter and Associates, Inc; 2010.
5. *2010 Medical Directorship and On-Call Compensation Survey.* Englewood, CO: Medical Group Management Association; 2010.
6. *2010 Physician On-Call Pay Survey.* Atlanta, GA: Sullivan, Cotter and Associates, Inc; 2010.
7. Morris L. Advisory Opinion No. 08-16. Washington, DC: Office of Inspector General; October 7, 2008.

APPENDIX A
Resources

Coker Group. *Reimbursement Management: Improving the Success and Profitability of Your Medical Practice.* Chicago: American Medical Association; 2011.

Topics include insurance basics, negotiation process, coding basics, back-office processes, billing and reimbursement, and the role of information technology.

Daigrepont JP. *Automating the Medical Record.* 2nd ed. Chicago: American Medical Association; 2004.

Topics include the electronic medical record (EMR), computer technology, networks, conversion to an EMR, the influence of Health Insurance Portability and Accountability Act (HIPAA), and vendor relations.

Coker Group. *Starting, Buying, and Owning a Medical Practice.* 3rd ed. Chicago: American Medical Association; 2011.

Topics include tax and licensing requirements; operational policy, procedures, and processing; , personnel management, medical record keeping, financial asset considerations, revenue cycle management, information technology, risk management, marketing strategies; physician alignment, employment, practice acquisition, equity structuring, diversification, practice mergers, and planning processes.

Coker Group. *Assessing and Improving Billing and Collections.* Chicago: American Medical Association; 2000.

Topics include self-assessment, patient encounters, and assessments of the billing process.

Coker Group. *Financial Management of the Medical Practice.* 3rd ed. Chicago: American Medical Association; 2011.

Topics include financial planning, budgeting processes, internal controls for collections, fraud prevention, and flash reports.

Reiboldt JM, Hunter CW. *Beyond Disengagement: Recreating the Physician Practice.* Chicago: American Medical Association; 2001.

Topics include financial, strategic, and operational issues and disengagement.

Stanley KB, Reeves CS, Coker Group. *Managing the Medical Practice.* 2nd ed. Chicago: American Medical Association; 2003.

Topics include personnel management, financial management, facility and operations management, purchasing, marketing, and risk management.

Stanley KB. *Personnel Management in the Medical Practice.* 2nd ed. Chicago: American Medical Association; 2002.

Topics include management issues, motivational techniques, communication styles, and team building.

APPENDIX B

South Atlanta Orthopedic and Physical Therapy, Inc

Appendix B provides an example of a valuation sample operating results of a fictional practice named "South Atlanta Orthopedic and Physical Therapy, Inc." These hypothetical financial statements reveal where an appraiser may gather information in a real appraisal.

The figures used in this example are not from any actual medical practice—the names have not been changed. This is a fictional example. Any similarity to any medical practice or otherwise is completely happenstance. However, the numbers that have been used are close to what a physician practice with a physical therapy (PT) component would resemble.

This book this is not meant to be a "mini-MBA." It does not delve into the volumes upon volumes of information about appraisals and appraisal theory, and it is not directed toward someone with a doctorate degree. It is meant for someone who has a general understanding of financial management, accounting, and finance, and the financial examples have been laid out accordingly.

Overview of the Practice

South Atlanta Orthopedic and Physical Therapy, LLC, is a two-physician orthopedic practice that specializes in sports medicine. In addition to orthopedic services, it also provides an in-house PT suite with a full range of free weights, body building equipment, and cardiovascular equipment; a therapeutic pool; and other exercise equipment. In addition to the physician providers, two full-time physical therapists work in the PT center. The staff breakdown is as follows:

TABLE B-1 Overview of South Atlanta Orthopedic and Physical Therapy, LLC

Position	Full-Time Equivalent	Individual Compensation*	Total Compensation
Physical Therapist	2	$50,000	$100,000
Office Manager	1	$38,000	$38,000
Patient Service Representative (PSR)	2	$23,000	$46,000
Billing	1	$30,000	$30,000
Registered Nurse/X-Ray Technician	2	$33,000	$66,000
Medical Assistant	1.25	$28,000	$35,000
Total Staff	9		$315,000

*Approximate compensation

The practice owns a considerable amount of PT and medical equipment (including an x-ray machine) but not its own facility. The space is leased, and the rent is assumed to be fair market value for the area. The practice has operated in its current capacity for approximately nine years, and while it has offered the same services for this period, it has recently upgraded some of its equipment and invested in some more technologically advanced PT equipment. The practice has had stable operations over its history. Both of the physicians are somewhat entrenched in the community and are expected to remain on as employees of the larger group. The practice has financed most of its growth in purchasing equipment through the acquisition of debt; however, it presently has an excellent credit rating through its lenders.

Currently, Atlanta Orthopedic Physicians, PA (AOP), is considering the purchase of a 100% interest in the practice. AOP is a large orthopedic group consisting of more than 275 orthopedic physicians (not including non-physician providers). In addition to orthopedic services, AOP provides PT and a host of other ancillary services (including imaging, laboratory, etc). AOP's operations are centered in Atlanta, Georgia, but it provides services throughout the southeastern United States, with practices in Louisiana, Mississippi, Alabama, Georgia, Tennessee, South Carolina, and North Carolina.

The effective date of this valuation is as of January 1, 2011.

Financial Statements for South Atlanta Orthopedics and Physical Therapy, LLC

EXHIBIT B-1—Income Statement for Last Four Years

South Atlanta Orthopedics and Physical Therapy, LLC Profit and Loss Statement for the Fiscal Year January 1 through December 31								
	FY 2010	**Percent to Net Revenue**	**FY 2009**	**Percent to Net Revenue**	**FY 2008**	**Percent to Net Revenue**	**FY 2007**	**Percent to Net Revenue**
Revenue								
Fees From Medical Operations	$3,689,023	156.25%	S3,347,571	161.29%	$3,218,818.06	163.93%	$3,008,241.18	161.29%
Less: Discounts and Reimbursements	($1,328,048)	-56.25%	($1,272,077)	-61.29%	($1,255,339.04)	-63.93%	($1,143,131.65)	–61.29%
Net Revenue	$2,360,975	100.00%	$2,075,494	100.00%	$1,963,479	100.00%	$1,865,110	100.00%
Expenses								
Personnel Expenses								
Physician Benefits	$155,656	6.59%	$148,244	7.14%	$141,185	7.19%	$133,193	7.14%
Physician Compensation	$695,125	29.44%	$662,024	31.90%	$630,499	32.11%	$594,810	31.89%
Staff Benefits	$75,025	3.18%	$71,452	3.44%	$68,050	3.47%	$64,198	3.44%
Staff Salary	$315,151	13.35%	$300,144	14.46%	$285,851	14.56%	$269,671	14.46%
Total Personnel Expenses	$1,240,957	52.56%	$1,181,864	56.94%	$1,125,585	54.23%	$1,061,872	51.16%
General & Administrative (G&A) Expenses								
Advertising and Promotion	$35,252	1.49%	$32,337	1.56%	$35,152	1.79%	$30,362	1.63%
Amortization	$14,500	0.61%	$14,500	0.70%	$8,561	0.44%	$7,321	0.39%
Automotive	$15,325	0.65%	$13,352	0.64%	$10,520	0.54%	$8,525	0.46%
Continuing Medical Education	$4,985	0.21%	$3,352	0.16%	$3,362	0.17%	$3,299	0.18%

South Atlanta Orthopedics and Physical Therapy, LLC Profit and Loss Statement for the Fiscal Year January 1 through December 31								
	FY 2010	Percent to Net Revenue	FY 2009	Percent to Net Revenue	2008	Percent to Net Revenue	2007	Percent to Net Revenue
Depreciation	$75,895	3.21%	$50,325	2.42%	$45,935	2.34%	$50,436	2.70%
Dues and Subscriptions	$4,567	0.19%	$4,012	0.19%	$40,012	2.04%	$38,765	2.08%
Insurance	$55,011	2.33%	$57,023	2.75%	$55,252	2.81%	$54,358	2.91%
Interest Expense	$75,898	3.21%	$55,025	2.65%	$50,253	2.56%	$50,253	2.69%
Laundry	$1,255	0.05%	$2,025	0.10%	$2,033	0.10%	$2,145	0.12%
Leased Equipment	$4,035	0.17%	$4,035	0.19%	$6,736	0.34%	$6,735	0.36%
Outside Services	$4,585	0.19%	$3,385	0.16%	$22,265	1.13%	$1,657	0.09%
Payroll Expense	$8,211	0.35%	$8,025	0.39%	$7,598	0.39%	$7,435	0.40%
Professional Fees	$85,426	3.62%	$34,554	1.66%	$35,425	1.80%	$33,452	1.79%
Professional Liability	$155,252	6.58%	$98,058	4.72%	$97,025	4.94%	$96,025	5.15%
Rental Expense	$135,000	5.72%	$128,571	6.19%	$122,449	6.24%	$116,618	6.25%
Supplies—Computer	$5,688	0.24%	$4,658	0.22%	$3,555	0.18%	$3,758	0.20%
Supplies—Laboratory	$80,122	3.39%	$78,025	3.76%	$77,001	3.92%	$76,050	4.08%
Supplies—Medical	$135,002	5.72%	$122,589	5.91%	$120,569	6.14%	$119,985	6.43%
Supplies—Office	$20,133	0.85%	$19,857	0.96%	$19,235	0.98%	$19,777	1.06%
Travel and Entertainment	$7,022	0.30%	$5,552	0.27%	$5,032	0.26%	$4,998	0.27%
Utilities	$52,023	2.20%	$54,023	2.60%	$53,252	2.71%	$52,025	2.79%
Total G&A Expenses	$975,187	41.30%	$793,283	38.22%	$821,222	41.82%	$783,979	42.03%
Total Expenses	$2,216,144	93.87%	$1,975,147	95.17%	$1,946,807	99.15%	$1,845,851	98.97%
Net Income Before Taxes	$144,831	6.13%	$100,347	4.83%	$16,672	0.85%	$19,258	1.03%

EXHIBIT B-2—Balance Sheet for Last Four Years

	South Atlanta Orthopedics and Physical Therapy, LLC Balance Sheet			
	FY 2010	FY 2009	FY 2008	FY 2007
Assets				
Current Assets				
Cash (Money Market Account)	$12,502	$14,300	$10,050	$9,580
Accounts Receivable	$225,898	$200,123	$215,023	$203,323
Total Current Assets	$238,400	$214,423	$225,073	$212,903
Long-Term Assets				
Property, Plant and Equipment	$753,252	$717,383	$650,130	$663,261
Accumulated Depreciation	$102,589	$85,012	$93,946	$90,333
Total Long-Term Assets	$650,663	$632,371	$556,184	$572,928
Total Assets	**$889,063**	**$846,794**	**$781,257**	**$785,831**
Liabilities				
Current Liabilities				
Accounts Payable	$5,252	$5,252	$4,235	$5,674
Short-Term Debt	$15,250	$20,120	$14,757	$13,654
Total Current Liabilities	$20,502	$25,372	$18,992	$19,328
Long-Term Liabilities				
Long-Term Debt				
Eastern Bank Loan	$455,005	$470,132	$454,021	$458,923
Central Bank Line of Credit	$55,121	$12,525	$0	$0
Total Long-Term Liabilities	$510,126	$482,657	$454,021	$458,923
Total Liabilities	$530,628	$508,029	$473,013	$478,251
Equity	$337,933	$313,393	$289,252	$288,252
Total Liabilities and Equity	**$889,063**	**$846,794**	**$781,257**	**$785,831**

EXHIBIT B-3—Adjusted Expenses

Year	FY 2007	FY 2008	FY 2009	FY 2010	Average
Actual Expenses	**$2,216,144**	**$1,975,147**	**$1,946,807**	**$1,845,851**	**$1,995,987**
Expense Adjustments					
Backed-Out					
Physician Benefits	($155,656)	($148,244)	($141,185)	($133,193)	($144,569)
Physician Compensation	($695,125)	($662,024)	($630,499)	($594,810)	($645,614)
Amortization	($14,500)	($14,500)	($8,561)	($7,321)	($11,221)
Automotive	($15,325)	($13,352)	($10,520)	($8,525)	($11,931)
Continuing Medical Education	($4,985)	($3,352)	($3,362)	($3,299)	($3,750)
Depreciation	($75,895)	($50,325)	($45,935)	($50,436)	($55,648)
Outside Services	$0	$0	($22,265)	$0	($5,566)
Professional Fees	($85,426)	$0	$0	$0	($21,357)
Travel and Entertainment	($7,022)	($5,552)	($5,032)	($4,998)	($5,651)
Total Backed-Out Expenses	($1,053,934)	($897,349)	($867,358)	($802,582)	($905,306)
Added Expenses					
Physician Benefits	$141,674	$137,547	$133,541	$129,651	$135,603
Physician Compensation	$708,368	$687,736	$667,705	$648,257	$678,016
Outside Services	$0	$0	$2,500	$0	$625
Professional Services	$35,000	$0	$0	$0	$8,750
Total Expenses Added	$885,042	$825,283	$803,746	$777,908	$822,995
Total Expense Adjustments	($168,892)	($72,066)	($63,613)	($24,674)	($82,311)
Adjusted Expenses	**$2,047,252**	**$1,903,082**	**$1,883,194**	**$1,821,178**	**$1,913,676**

EXHIBIT B-4—Performance Summary for Last Four Years

Year	FY 2010	FY 2009	FY 2008	FY 2007	Average
Revenue	**$2,360,975**	**$2,075,494**	**$1,963,479**	**$1,865,110**	**$1,968,027**
Expenses	**$2,216,144**	**$1,975,147**	**$1,946,807**	**$1,845,851**	**$1,922,602**
Percent to Total	93.87%	95.17%	99.15%	98.97%	97.69%
Profit	$144,831	$100,347	$16,672	$19,258	$45,426
Adjusted Expenses	**$2,047,252**	**$1,903,082**	**$1,883,194**	**$1,821,178**	**$1,869,151**
Percent to Total	86.71%	91.69%	95.91%	97.64%	94.98%
Adjusted Profit	$313,723	$172,412	$80,285	$43,932	$98,876
Revenue to Expense Correlation				0.9390	
Revenue to Adjusted Expense Correlation				0.9473	

EXHIBIT B-5—Balance Sheet Adjustments

	FY 2010 Balance Sheet	Adjustments	FY 2010 Balance Sheet Adjusted
Assets			
Current Assets			
Cash (Money Market Account)	$12,502	$0	$12,502
Accounts Receivable (1)	$225,898	($75,898)	$150,000
Total Current Assets	$238,400	($75,898)	$162,502
Long-Term Assets			
Property, Plant and Equipment (2)	$753,252	($75,325)	$677,927
Accumulated Depreciation	$102,589	$0	$0
Total Long-Term Assets	$650,663	($75,325)	$677,927
Total Assets	**$889,063**		**$840,429**
Liabilities			
Current Liabilities			
Accounts Payable	$5,252	$0	$5,252
Short-Term Debt	$15,250	$0	$15,250
Total Current Liabilities	$20,502	$0	$20,502
Long-Term Liabilities			
Long-Term Debt			
Eastern Bank Loan	$372,609	$0	$372,609
Central Bank Line of Credit	$55,121	$0	$55,121
Total Long-Term Liabilities	$427,730	$0	$427,730
Total Liabilities	**$448,232**	**$0**	**$448,232**
Equity	**$420,329**	**$0**	**$420,329**
Total Liabilities and Equity	**$889,063**	**$0**	**$889,063**

(1) Discounted to fair collectible value

(2) Discount based on fair market value of furniture and equipment

Market Analysis Data

Publicly Traded Market Data

The following companies were used when completing the guideline publicly traded company method. The companies below are all publicly traded companies (their stock ticker symbol is listed beside their name). A brief description of the company and what it does have been provided.

- National Physical Therapy (NPT)
  - NPT provides PT services in 35 states across the country and in Mexico and Canada. It employs no physicians. The majority of NPT's locations are in the eastern, mid-Atlantic states, and the Midwest; it has no presence in the western United States.
- Physical Therapy Associates (PTA)
  - PTA provides PT services in 10 states, mostly in the Southwest to mid-Southern states. It is focused on rural areas and cities with populations of 50,000 or less. It owns very little of the real estate it occupies, and it does not employ its physicians, but it does employ all other providers (eg, physical therapists, etc).
- Orthopedics of America (OA)
  - OA is an orthopedic medical practice management company. It is based in the Northwest, and the majority of its services is provided to practices in Washington, Oregon, Idaho, Montana, and Canada (although it does have a minimal presence in California). It owns no real estate associated with its operations. Its primary line of business is associated with providing management services to smaller orthopedic practices (1-5 physicians). The services that are provided range from employing the staff to billing and collections; the services are provided via a contract basis.
- National Ortho (NO)
  - NO is a nationwide provider of orthopedic and allied care services ranging from PT to podiatry and surgical care services. NO is located in all 50 states and in Puerto Rico, Europe, Mexico, and Canada. These locations consist of full-service sites that provide "one-stop" physician and ancillary services to sites that just provide one service or another (ie, surgical center only, PT center only, etc). A major entrance into the western US market was made in 2001 with the purchase of StrengthPac, a provider of PT services. It owns approximately half of its real estate through a subsidiary venture, Healthcare Facility Managers, Inc (this information is not included on its financial statements).

- Northern Health Associates (NHA)
  - NHA provides orthopedic management and PT services in Illinois, Indiana, Ohio, and Kentucky. This company is fairly new, having only operated for two and one-half years.
- Sector: Healthcare Providers
- Industry: Healthcare

Following is a summary of the guideline public companies' operations:

EXHIBIT B-6—Guideline Public Data Company

Public Company Data								
Public Company	As Of	Revenue	EBITDA	Shares Outstanding	Market Capitalization	Invested Capital	MVIC/ Revenue	MVIC/EBITDA
NPT	1/1/2011	$102,325,455	$19,568,467	100,555,232	$2,287,631,528.00	$105,858,632	1.03	5.41
PTA	1/1/2011	$77,258,952	$7,035,111	13,585,653	$102,979,249.74	$102,589,325	1.33	14.58
OA	1/1/2011	$45,895,235	$8,987,025	15,252,222	$149,624,297.82	$32,577,789	0.71	3.62
NO	1/1/2011	$195,556,216	$37,632,141	55,200,011	$1,796,760,358.05	$232,527,002	1.19	6.18
NHA	1/1/2011	$39,958,567	$5,552,325	7,000,111	$7,210,114.33	$45,656,578	1.14	8.22

High		$195,556,216	$37,632,141	$100,555,232	$2,287,631,528	$232,527,002	1.33	14.58
Low		$39,958,567	$5,552,325	$7,000,111	$7,210,114	$32,577,789	0.71	3.62
Median		$77,258,952	$8,987,025	$15,252,222	$149,624,298	$102,589,325	1.14	6.18

EBITDA: earnings before interest, taxes, depreciation, and amortization

MVIC: market value of invested capital

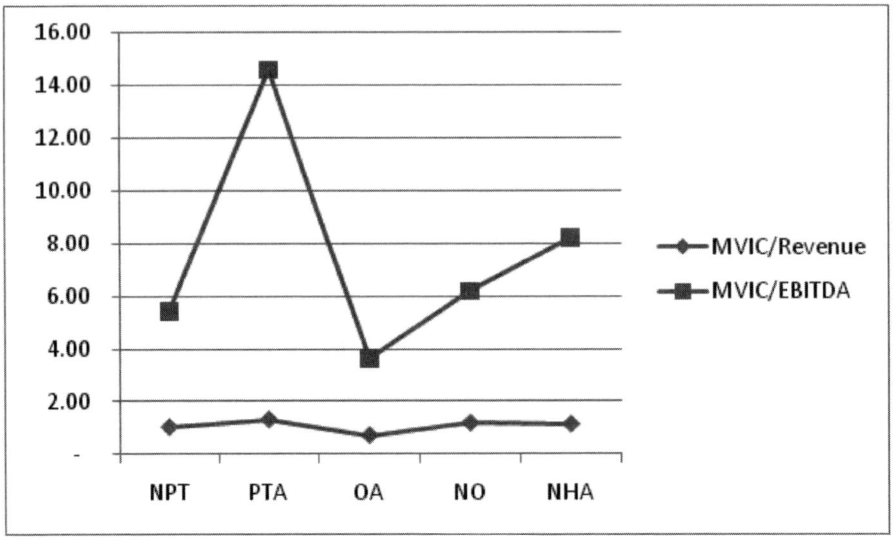

FIGURE B-1 Graphical Representation of Stock Prices

Previously Acquired Company Data

- Orthopedics Associates of Kentucky (OAK)
  - OAK provided orthopedic management services throughout Kentucky and Ohio to approximately 25 different orthopedic practices ranging in size of one physician to five. In June 2001, NHA purchased 100% of OAK, which consisted of a stock and debt transaction.
- National Orthopedic Consultants (NOC)
  - NOC provided a wide range of orthopedic and PT services across the Midwest. At the time of its purchase, it employed approximately 42 full-time providers at over 15 different locations. A 100% interest of NOC was purchased by NO in September 2009.
- Physical Therapy Services of California (PTSC)
  - PTSC provided PT services in an around Sacramento, California. It was purchased in 2008 by California-based StrengthPac, Inc, to expand its services into the northern California area.
- Rehabilitative Associates of New Orleans (RAN)
  - RAN had two locations in the greater New Orleans area. A 100% interest was purchased in the beginning of this year, which included a pure equity purchase. The acquirer was Southern Rehab (SORB), Dallas, Texas.

- StrengthPac (SP)
  - SP provided PT services in the western half of the United States, with the majority of its clinics in California, Arizona, Nevada, and Colorado. It was purchased by NO to expand its services into the western United States.
- Health Source (HS)
  - HS managed a number of orthopedic practices in the eastern United States, ranging from New York to Florida. At its peak in the 2000s, HS managed over 390 practices; however, this figure had decreased considerably by the time it was acquired by American Physician Managers (AMPM). This acquisition was made in 2010 for 100% equity interest.

The following is a summary of the information from these transactions:

EXHIBIT B-7—Previous Transactional Information

Target	Date	Revenue	Net Income	Total Assets	MVIC	MVIC/ EBITDA	MVIC/ Revenue
PTSC	7/1/2008	$9,935,456	$1,244,662	$6,252,535	$5,663,210	4.55	0.57
SP	4/1/2009	$32,925,078	$5,192,485	$29,024,361	$28,974,069	5.58	0.88
OAK	6/1/2010	$404,478	$44,512	$334,558	$279,090	6.27	0.69
HS	5/1/2010	$25,180,106	$4,490,358	$19,992,536	$19,892,284	4.43	0.79
NOC	9/1/2009	$595,901	$91,755	$552,520	$542,270	5.91	0.91
RAN	1/1/2010	$666,031	$172,928	$746,212	$672,691	3.89	1.01
High		$32,925,078	$5,192,485	$29,024,361	$28,974,069	6.27	1.01
Low		$404,478	$44,512	$334,558	$279,090	3.89	0.57
Median		$5,300,743	$708,795	$3,499,374	$3,167,951	5.07	0.84

MVIC: market value of invested capital

EBITDA: earnings before interest, taxes, depreciation, and amortization

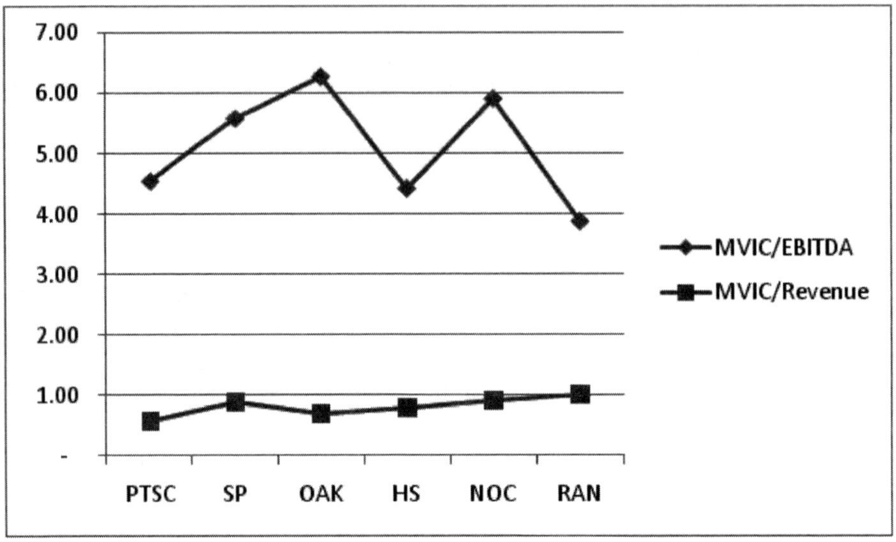

FIGURE B-2 Transaction Multiples

APPENDIX C
Informational Sites and World Wide Web Research

There are literally thousands of sites providing information on general appraisal topics as well as health care appraisal topics. This appendix provides a number of useful sites. Some of these sites are free (but often plagued with pop-up ads); some are a combination of free and subscription sites; and some are outright membership sites. It can cost a small fortune to subscribe to every subscription and membership site, so it is best to make use of the free sites (and deal with the advertisements) and be more discriminating when choosing pay sites. Also included in this appendix are a number of related sites that may prove invaluable to appraisers.

General Search Engines

Various items can be found by using general search engines. They serve as a good way to begin any search. A few search engines perform meta-searches that compile searches of smaller engines or that sort unrelated material and return only the most pertinent information from each search. A good general rule is to conduct a search in more than one search engine to obtain a comprehensive listing on the Internet.

www.google.com
Google is a great search engine and widely used for business searches.

www.yahoo.com
Yahoo is a commonly used search engine.

www.lycos.com
Lycos will return a comprehensive search of related sites and information.

www.search.msn.com
This link is to the search engine Bing and to Microsoft news.

www.hotbot.com
HotBot is a meta-search engine that filters nonrelated subjects from smaller engine searches and displays the most pertinent ones.

www.go.com or www.infoseek.com
This search engine from Disney Interactive Media Group is much like Yahoo. It is powered by Yahoo for searching the Web.

www.metacrawler.com
Metacrawler compiles several search engines and sorts each search into categories.

www.dogpile.com
Dogpile™ searches Google, Yahoo, and Bing and filters nonrelated material to provide the most useful information from each search.

www.ask.com
With ask.com, the user types in a question and ask.com returns Web sites that can answer the question.

www.search.com
This search engine compiles searchable databases from many different sources on the Web.

www.business.com
This Web site compiles hundreds of company Web sites and provides related links to more companies with similar functions.

www.findarticles.com
This database of articles from CBS Business Network can provide insight into almost any search as well as links to related material.

News and Business Sources

It is imperative that the appraiser be well-informed about current issues in the marketplace, especially when performing valuations. The following sites are some news sources for general business. This list is broad and may not contain every possible site, but it will provide the health care appraiser with a wealth of market information.

www.wsj.com
A business news periodical, the *Wall Street Journal* has nonmember and member information.

www.economist.com
This is an online version of *The Economist,* a journal providing daily information on business and economic events.

www.ceoexpress.com
CEO Express is an excellent resource providing comprehensive information about and links to US and world news.

www.cnbc.com
This is the CNBC Web site for financial news and data.

www.bloomberg.com
Bloomberg provides updated business news and financial information.

www.capitaliq.com
Capital IQ provides very useful data and analytics for financial professionals.

www.money.cnn.com
CNN financial news is a link to *CNNMoney*, *Money,* and *Fortune* magazines.

www.cfo.com
This is the link to *CFO* magazine.

www.hoovers.com
Hoovers™ is a member Web site that allows users to research any type of information on thousands of publicly traded companies.

www.finance.yahoo.com
This Yahoo site can provide quick and easily accessible information to most publicly traded companies.

www.foxnews.com
Fox News online offers current news and world events.

www.nytimes.com
This is link to *The New York Times* Web site.

www.usatoday.com
This is the link to *USA Today*.

www.economy.com/dismal
This is an economics site that uses government statistics to provide economic profiles, both as historical and forecasted, for different areas of the United States.

www.rollcall.com
A biweekly newspaper, *Roll Call* is considered a must read for insiders in Congress.

www.thehill.com
The Hill is a useful newspaper for those looking to stay current with the news on Capitol Hill.

www.compustat.com
Capital IQ Compustat serves as a leading resource for in-depth financial information on publicly traded companies in the United States and around the world.

Health Care Information and News Sites

In addition to being current on general news, anyone valuing a health care entity must know current information and where to find it, including archival press releases and articles pertaining to various sectors of the industry. The following sites are excellent resources.

www.mpmnetwork.com
This is the link to the *Journal of Medical Practice Management,* a health care office management publication for administrators.

www.uoworks.com
Unique Opportunities provides resources for physicians, including recruiting resources.

www.webmd.com
WebMD keeps visitors up-to-date on current and recent health issues.

www.medicaleconomics.com
This link provides current news and financial information from the *Medical Economics* magazine.

www.bcbshealthissues.com
At the Blue Cross and Blue Shield Association's Web site, visitors can search for information on health-related issues and conditions.

www.forbes.com/healthcare
Daily news is provided to members of the *Forbes Magazine* online.

www.nih.gov/news
This site from the National Institutes of Health provides health information and recent news and events in the world of medicine.

www.reutershealth.com
This membership Web site to Reuters Health provides current information on global pharmaceutical, medical, and consumer health-related issues.

www.worldhealthnews.harvard.edu
This is a weekly journal from the Harvard School of Public Health.

www.healthleadersmedia.com
Visitors can access updates, press releases, and archival searches from *HealthLeaders* magazine.

Health Care Sites and Associations

Many sites on the Internet can provide valuable information to appraisers and researchers on new advances in medical specialties. They offer links to a wealth of current trends and news for hospitals and clinical physicians alike. Following is a short list of organizations that can serve as a springboard to those interested in finding specific information on different health care specialties.

www.cancer.org
The American Cancer Society has links and information about cancer and support groups for families.

www.mayoclinic.com
The Mayo Clinic Web site has information and links for health conditions and questions.

www.ncqa.org
This link to the National Commission on Quality Assurance can provide information on current issues as well as links to related sites.

www.ahcancal.org
The American Health Care Association provides informational links and research about frail, elderly, and disabled Americans.

www.chipmedicaid.org
This Web site offers links, research, and other information pertaining to child health care programs.

www.asco.org
This is the American Society of Clinical Oncology Web site. This free membership Web site provides information about cancer research, care, and prevention, and links to more information regarding public policy and guidelines.

www. heart.org
The American Heart Association offers the user information on cardiovascular diseases and stroke, with a focus on preventive care and education, with links to related organizations.

www.rsna.org
The Radiologist Society of North America is a nonprofit professional organization for radiologists.

www.naph.org
The National Association of Public Hospital and Health Systems collectively represents safety net hospitals and health systems. Association publications deal with issues of quality, community health, chronic conditions, disparities, and finance.

Government Sites

Not to be overlooked, government Web sites can also provide much helpful information on all types of issues. They can provide general information, including statistics, and specific information about regulations that govern the administration and organization of health care as well as general business information that appraisers should consider when evaluating companies.

www.cdc.gov
Visitors to the US Centers for Disease Control and Prevention can find information and statistics on various diseases and health conditions.

www.hhs.gov
This is the Department of Health and Human Services Web site. Users can find information on its 11 operating divisions, including those on health insurance, research, public health, food and drug safety, and Medicare fraud.

www.nih.gov
The National Institutes of Health is part of the Department of Health and Human Services and is the nation's medical research agency. Links to each of the institutes provide valuable resources.

www.nlm.nih.gov
The National Library of Medicine Web site links to the world's largest medical library.

www.fedstats.gov
Fedstats offers a full range of official statistical information produced by the federal government, with searching and linking capabilities to more than 100 agencies that provide data and trend information.

www.usa.gov
This link is the official Web portal of the US government and offers information on all aspects of the government.

www.sec.gov
This is the Web site of the US Securities and Exchange Commission. It is helpful for researchers who want to stay current on market regulations.

www.cms.gov
This is the site for the Centers for Medicare and Medicaid Services. It has information on subjects relating to Medicare and Medicaid issues and initiatives.

Valuation Resources

Many World Wide Web sites provide great resources for those who seek to value or appraise companies. Often an appraiser must gather market data along with data from past mergers and acquisitions. The following sites can provide data and a starting place for searches to find comparative analysis and information. Sometimes these sites charge a fee for their service; however, the fees are worth the cost for anyone looking to accurately appraise the value of a business.

www.valuationresources.com
This site offers business valuation information. Designed to be a comprehensive resource guide for business appraisers, it provides links to resources for people interested in business valuation and industry information.

www.appraisers.org
This is the official site of the American Society of Appraisers.

www.bvmarketdata.com
BVMarketData.com^{SM} contains searchable databases and reports and links the user to information on purchases and mergers and acquisitions that are helpful to business appraisers.

www.bizminer.com
Biz Miner provides financial analysis and market data on thousands of companies, including hard-to-find industry analysis.

www.levinassociates.com
For a fee, the user can find information such as health care mergers and acquisitions and financial analysis from Irving Levin Associates, Inc.

www.marketresearch.com
Market Research offers information on products, trends, regions, demographics, industries, and companies from more than 700 research publishers.

www.bvlibrary.com
The Web site for Business Valuation Resources is a solid guide and provides searchable databases for those interested in valuations and appraisals.

www.appraisalfoundation.org
The Appraisal Foundation is a nonprofit organization and a good starting point for business appraisers who are looking for standard valuation methods and techniques.

www.finweb.com
Financial Web is helpful when comparing stock prices for more than one day at a time. Archival information on historical prices and other market data are available.

www.djindexes.com
The Dow Jones Indexes Web site can be a basis for beginning a business search.

www.morningstar.com
Morningstar provides industry-leading data on investment offerings.

GLOSSARY

A

amortization The recovery of an expense item over a period based on the economic value and life of the *asset*.

appraisal and valuation The term *appraisal* has been referred to as the overall process of review, while a *valuation* is the actual determination of monetary worth. Within the context of this publication, the terms are synonymous.

asset-based approach Estimating the reproduction costs of assets of the practice. *Tangible* and *intangible assets* are valued individually on a going-concern basis, and then accumulated to derive total value.

asset The economic resource of the practice (ie, property and equipment, cash, and accounts receivable).

B

book value *Asset* minus *liability*. This is generally an accounting term that reflects an owner's *equity*.

C

capital Money accumulated for investment or retirement purposes.

capitalization A process of converting net income that results from period-to-period operations into a lump sum present value. Rates for such capitalization are normally called *CAP rates*.

capitalization rate Generally calculated as the *discount rate* less long-term growth ($r_e - g$).

capitation A method of reimbursement under *managed care* plans by which professional providers receive a fixed fee per member per month for each of the plan's enrollees who have selected them as their primary care physician.

cash flow The actual results of practice operations (cash receipts minus disbursements) without consideration of noncash items such as *depreciation* and interest.

comparative value Value based on recent selling prices of area practices similar to the one for sale.

D

depreciation Depreciation is the process of allocating the cost of an *asset* to the periods of benefit. Accumulated depreciation is total *depreciation* change on an asset since its acquisition.

designated health services A list of 10 specific entities, as identified by federal legislation, that provide health care services. Referrals to specific services are placed under strict controls for preventing private inurement, private benefit, and other Medicare fraud and abuse violations.

diagnosis-related group (DRG) The DRG was developed for Medicare in the early 1980s as part of its prospective payment system. This schedule reimburses hospitals a flat fee based on diagnosis; surgical procedure (if applicable); patient sex, age, and medical status; and complications for approximately 500 surgical procedures and diagnoses. Some commercial carriers and *Health Maintenance Organizations* implemented their own DRG schedules for inpatient and outpatient surgical procedures. Medicare is still using DRG reimbursements, although they have been updated since the inception of the program.

discounted cash flow valuation (DCF) Present value of forecasted *cash flow* plus present value of terminal or residual value equals the current value of core operations of the practice.

discounting This is a process of projecting present value of the entitlement to receive money in the future, reducing the worth of the dollar by certain percentages for risk and minority interest to its present value.

discount rate The *capitalization rate* applied to convert future income streams to arrive at today's present value.

discount A process of adjusting for risk.

E

EBITDA Acronym for earnings before interest, taxes, depreciation, and amortization. Various forms of this may include EBIT (earnings before interest and taxes), EBT, and EAT (earnings after taxes).

equity Ownership interest.

F

fair market value Price (value) negotiated at arm's length between a willing buyer and a willing seller, each acting rationally in his or her own self-interest.

fee-for-service (FFS) A system of payment in which payment is made to physicians, hospitals, and other providers based on services rendered to the patient.

G

going concern An ongoing operating business enterprise.

going concern value The value of a business enterprise that is expected to continue to operate into the future. The intangible elements of going concern value result from factors such as having a trained workforce, an operational plant, and the necessary licenses, systems, and procedures in place.

H

health maintenance organization (HMO) An organization responsible for providing or arranging the provision of comprehensive health care services on a prepayment basis to voluntarily enrolled persons within a designated population. The providers are aligned and under contract with the plan for a fixed and periodic payment. When an HMO purchases an institution that delivers health care, this model is fully integrated because both financing and delivery of care are provided to the enrolled members.

I

income approach to valuation Present worth analysis of anticipated future monetary benefits. Estimated future *cash flow* is converted to present value based on an appropriate *discount rate* or rate of return.

independent practice association (IPA) Entity formed by physicians, sometimes with another health care provider, such as a hospital. Generally, it is formed to provide a vehicle for effective contracting with *managed care* purchasers. IPAs contract with HMOs, *Preferred Provider Organizations,* and other managed care companies to provide professional medical services. They differ from group practices in that IPA practices remain independent. Also known as *independent physician associations.*

intangible asset Non-tangible asset such as customer lists, goodwill, securities, contracts, etc.

integrated delivery system (IDS) Alliances between health care providers including hospitals, sole practitioners, and group practices. Usually, it is designed for providing overall delivery of health care to the patient.

invested capital (IC) method The sum of *equity* and debt in a business enterprise.

investment (or strategic) value The value of an asset for specific users reflecting the utility and profitability to an enterprise.

L

lack of marketability The absence of a ready or existing market for the sale of the practice.

liability Debt due and payable, such as accounts payable, taxes, and notes payable. Current liabilities are those that are due within a short time, usually one year.

liquidation value The anticipated revenue from disposing of equipment under a forced or semi-forced condition.

liquidity The convertibility of an asset to cash.

M

managed care A system of financing and providing health care services to a defined group of individuals. Managed care plans provide alliances of providers for thc cxpress purpose of containing costs, promoting wellness, and appropriate use of services by its members. Managed care organizations are often *HMOs, PPOs,* and *IPAs.*

management service organization (MSO) An organization formed to provide a cross section of business functions, primarily for administrative management services for physician practices. However, sometimes the primary purpose is for *managed care* contracting. MSOs may also be structured to purchase physician practices and conduct administrative functions for other practices that may not be purchased. Services include accounting, billing, facility management, utilization review, consulting, computer software installation and support, professional fees, marketing, personnel services, etc. Financial arrangements of MSOs are varied. Ownership could include a combination of physicians, hospital, or each of them individually, or it may include a health care company and insurance company or private investors.

market approach to valuation Comparative analysis of prices paid for similar *assets* in the marketplace. Value is estimated by using the earnings capitalization multiples derived from sales of comparable medical practices or comparable publicly traded companies.

market value What a buyer or seller may expect to obtain for a practice in its related market.

Medicaid A federal program under the Social Security Administration that provides health care benefits to individuals who fall below the poverty level.

Medicare A federal program under the Social Security Administration that provides health insurance benefits to persons older than age 65 and others eligible for Social Security benefits.

Medicarc and Medicaid Fraud and Abuse Statute Law specifically outlining the illegality of a health care provider to knowingly and willfully alter, pay, solicit, or receive any remuneration directly or indirectly in return for the referral of a patient for the providing of any services paid for by Medicare or Medicaid.

minority interest Ownership of less than 50% control of the ownership of a practice.

P

physician-hospital organization (PHO) A health care model in which various providers form a network for *managed care* contracting. PHOs are modeled to include at least one hospital and a physician affiliation. The physicians may include both primary care and specialty practitioners. Usually, PHOs are separate entities with ownership and/or control divided between hospitals and physicians.

preferred provider organization (PPO) A plan or an organization that contracts with a specific and limited list of independent providers at a discounted fee-for-service in exchange for a channeled (or directed) patient base.

price to earnings (P/E) A typical ratio provided as a benchmark for companies. This ratio is typically used for public companies, as the price is readily known. The ratio is derived by dividing a company's stock price per share by the company's earnings.

proprietorship A privately owned business.

R

replacement cost The cost of a duplicate or equally viable substitute.

reproduction cost The cost of producing or constructing a new and identical replacement to the *asset.*

restrictive covenant An agreement (normally within the context of an employment or services contract) that restricts competition in that particular specialty. In a medical practice, it covers a physician who is agreeing not to compete in the geographical area after the sale of a practice or after leaving its employment. Also known as *noncompetition agreement.*

S

salvage value For accounting purposes, the estimated value of a depreciable *asset* at the end of its useful life.

Section 501(c)(3) Internal Revenue Code The code section that provides an exemption from federal income tax for not-for-profit organizations formed for charitable or community services.

single or multispecialty group practice Practices consisting of at least two physicians with the same or different medical specialties who typically share office space and other operating expenses.

sole proprietorship A business owned by a single individual.

Stark legislation Named for Congressman Forney "Pete" Stark (D), California, who previously chaired the House committee that addressed Medicare fraud and abuse violations. This legislation—typically called Stark I, II, and III—has specifically set guidelines for such violations.

T

tangible asset Property that can be specifically identified and is physical in nature (eg, equipment, land, cash, accounts receivable, buildings).

U

useful (service) life Refers to the period of expected usefulness of a tangible asset in the practice.

W

weighted average cost of capital (WACC) A method for determining the valuation of the invested capital (IC), ie, debt plus equity.

INDEX

Page numbers for figures and tables appear in italics.

B

C

D

G

H

I

J, K

L

M

N

O

P

W